SALT
IN MY
SOUL

AN
UNFINISHED
LIFE

MALLORY
SMITH

HAY HOUSE

Carlsbad, California • New York City
London • Sydney • New Delhi

Published in the United States by Spiegel & Grau, an imprint of Random House, a division of Penguin Random House LLC, New York.
www.penguinrandomhouse.com

Published in the United Kingdom by:
Hay House UK Ltd, Astley House, 33 Notting Hill Gate, London W11 3JQ
Tel: +44 (0)20 3675 2450; Fax: +44 (0)20 3675 2451; www.hayhouse.co.uk

Published in Australia by:
Hay House Australia Ltd, 18/36 Ralph St, Alexandria NSW 2015
Tel: (61) 2 9669 4299; Fax: (61) 2 9669 4144; www.hayhouse.com.au

Published in India by:
Hay House Publishers India, Muskaan Complex, Plot No.3, B-2,
Vasant Kunj, New Delhi 110 070
Tel: (91) 11 4176 1620; Fax: (91) 11 4176 1630; www.hayhouse.co.in

The information given in this book should not be treated as a substitute for professional medical advice; always consult a medical practitioner. Any use of information in this book is at the reader's discretion and risk. Neither the authors nor the publisher can be held responsible for any loss, claim or damage arising out of the use, or misuse, of the suggestions made, the failure to take medical advice or for any material on third-party websites.

A catalogue record for this book is available from the British Library.

Paperback ISBN: 978-1-78817-343-8
Ebook ISBN: 978-1-78817-348-3

Cover design by Lilli Colton
Book design by Susan Turner

Printed and bound by CPI Group (UK) Ltd, Croydon, CR0 4YY

I could title my memoir *Ode to Salt* since salt is part and parcel of the cystic fibrosis experience. Broken proteins lead to an imbalance of salt inside and out of the cells. If you kiss or lick the skin of a CF-er, you'll get a firsthand taste, literally, of how fundamental salt is to the disease. CF patients lose so much salt in our sweat that we can get water intoxication from drinking normal water unless we add salt to our water and our food. And salty water helps counteract some of the worst symptoms of the disease. I've noticed the healing effects of salt water since I was a little girl, swimming in the ocean in Southern California and on the many, many family trips we took to Hawaii for my health. I feel as if there's salt in my soul.

—*Mallory Smith*

Anyone who knew my daughter Mallory knew she kept a journal. She wrote during treatment, on vacation, when she should have been doing homework, in the hospital, in the middle of sleepless nights, at volleyball tournaments.

Once, when Mallory was in high school, after we had a big fight, she stormed into her room and started pounding on her laptop. From then on, I assumed her journal was a repository for her anger. So when Mal gave me the password before she went into transplant (she was afraid she "might not make it to the other side"), I imagined reading a recap of everything I'd ever done wrong as a mother. It was a terrifying thought.

I opened her journal the day of her memorial, thinking there might be something I could use when speaking about her. When I saw its scope—2,500 pages of her reflections over ten years—it became clear that Mallory had given me the most precious and unexpected gift a grieving mother could hope for.

The absence of any expression of anger toward me left me incredulous and grateful. But always thinking of other people's feelings was vintage Mallory. In the journal she left clear instructions for me not to let anyone else read the unedited version, so as not to hurt someone she might have railed against in a moment of anger, violate a friend's confidence, or expose the intimate details of her love life to her father or brother. She asked me to share the parts that might help others struggling with cystic fibrosis, loss, chronic illness, body image issues, depression, anxiety, or transplant.

Mallory's diagnosis of CF imposed a maturity on her and forced her to ask hard questions from a young age. The answers would lead her to develop a set of remarkable character traits, traits that helped her come to terms with her sickness and helped turn her into a strong, determined, talented young woman who motivated others as she found her way.

A three-sport varsity athlete in high school, Stanford University club volleyball player, and Phi Beta Kappa graduate, Mallory was passionate about the environment, channeling her interest into writing articles and producing radio programs. She wrote her first published book at the age of twenty-four, *The Gottlieb Native Garden: A California Love Story.*

But more important to Mallory than her accomplishments were her relationships. Her uncanny gift for cultivating friendships was especially remarkable in light of the torment of endless daily medical treatments, frequent hospitalizations, and frustrations caused by systemic hospital inefficiencies. Mallory never got to lead a normal life, but early on chose as her mantra "Live Happy," words she followed until her death.

Even at the end, tethered to an oxygen tank and round-the-clock IVs, Mallory exuded happiness as she fought for her life. She faced the overwhelming obstacles of a chronic, progressive illness with courage and grace. Healthcare providers saw her as the perfect patient, the poster child for compliance. But this façade of perfection masked a darker truth . . . a truth she shared only in the writing she left behind.

This is her story. These are her words.

—*Diane Shader Smith*

INTRODUCTION

I have big dreams and big goals. But also big limitations, which means I'll never reach the big goals unless I have the wisdom to recognize the chains that bind me. Only then will I be able to figure out a way to work within them instead of ignoring them or naively wishing they'll cease to exist. I'm on a perennial quest to find balance. Writing helps me do that.

To quote Neruda: *Tengo que acordarme de todos, recoger las briznas, los hilos del acontecer harapiento* (I have to remember everything, collect the wisps, the threads of untidy happenings). That line is ME. But my memory is slipping and that's one of the scariest aspects about all this. How can I tell my story, how can I create a narrative around my life, if I can't even remember the details?

But I do want to tell my story, and so I write.

I write because I want my parents to understand me. I write to leave something behind for them, for my brother Micah, for my boyfriend Jack, and for my extended family and friends, so I won't just end up as ashes scattered in the ocean and nothing else.

Curiously, the things I write in my journal are almost all bad: the letdowns, the uncertainties, the anxieties, the loneliness. The good stuff I keep in my head and heart, but that proves an unreliable way of holding on because time eventually steals all memories—and if it doesn't completely steal them, it distorts them, sometimes beyond recognition, or the emotional quality accompanying the moment just dissipates.

Many of the feelings I write about are too difficult to share while I'm alive, so I am keeping everything in my journal password-protected until the end. When I die I want my mom to edit these pages to ensure they are acceptable for publication— culling through years of writing, pulling together what will resonate, cutting references that might be hurtful. My hope is that my writing will offer insight for people living with, or loving someone with, chronic illness.

Cystic fibrosis is a chronic genetic illness that affects many parts of the body. It operates like this: A defective protein caused by the cystic fibrosis mutation interrupts the flow of salt in and out of cells, causing the mucus that's naturally present in healthy people to become dehydrated, thick, and viscous. This sticky mucus builds up in the lungs, pancreas, and other organs, causing problems with the respiratory, digestive, reproductive, endocrine, and other systems. In the lungs, the mucus creates a warm and welcoming environment for deadly bacteria like *Pseudomonas aeruginosa* and *Burkholderia cepacia*. The vicious cycle of infection, inflammation, and scarring that comes from the combination of viscous mucus and ineradicable bacteria leads to respiratory failure, the most common cause of death in cystic fibrosis patients.

It's progressive, with no cure, which means it gets worse over time. The rate of progression varies from patient to patient, and is often out of our control.

. . .

Cystic fibrosis is a disease that does a lot of taking—of dreams, of time, of travel, of friendships, of freedom, of potential, of plans, of lives.

Sitting in a hospital bed, I'm tempted to think about all the things that have been taken from me. More than that, it's easy to think about all the things I want for my future that might no longer be possible, the will-be-takens.

I was diagnosed at the age of three. As a kid, I made plans; I loved getting in bed at night because I had the opportunity to fantasize uninterrupted about whatever I was excited about. Some of what I thought about had to do with the future: where I would choose to live later in life, places I wanted to travel to, what I might be like as a teenager and then as an adult. Mostly, I envisioned other parts of the world—back then, anywhere was better than Los Angeles. The foreign always transcended the familiar. The unknown was brimming with possibility, while the known was full in a less satisfying way; like a big glass of a clumpy protein shake, you know it's good for you but it doesn't rock your world: daily routines, school days spent reading textbooks, long medical treatments I didn't want to do. As Dr. Seuss says, "You're off to great places! Today is your day! Your mountain is waiting, so . . . get on your way!" I believed wholeheartedly in those great places to come.

But for a CF patient, time is the meanest of forces. Just as water steadily erodes rock over the years, causing durable material to crumble with the invisible quality of slow change, my disease erodes the life blueprint I drew as a kid; with time, invisibly but surely, I grow decreasingly confident in the plans that I had etched in this mental map until it's hard to remember they were ever there. Occasionally, I'll remember with a smile the whimsical desires I had as a kid, and how tenaciously I fought for them—the dolphin research trip I desperately wanted to go on (never mind that we'd be living without electricity and I wouldn't be able to do treatment), my water polo team's trip to Hungary that I wished to go on without a parent. Now I chuckle because these fantasies were born out of a sense of entitlement, and I'm thankful to have outgrown that. How many kids, diseased or not, get to go on a research trip to Belize during high school? I couldn't go because I need electricity; most kids wouldn't have been able to go because it's indulgent and expensive.

The things I wanted were never material things, though. For the most part, I wished for a life lived honestly, to do good things, and to be happy. I wanted a career that, selflessly, would help people and, selfishly, would let me work in beautiful places and outdoors. I wanted beauty—not for me, but for my surroundings. Spending so much time trapped indoors has given me a deep appreciation for natural beauty.

A lot of the things I wished for have become reality. I'm incredibly grateful for the health I still have, the people who surround and support me, the time I got to spend at Stanford learning and growing into the person I am today, and the nourishing well of memories I'm able to draw from in times when the new memories I'm forming skew more negative than positive.

But I've also spent a lot more time than I would like wrestling demons, wasting precious energy suffering with problems derived from feeling like a victim. My life is constantly changing, and that's difficult. That's what CF does; like an earthquake, it constantly moves the ground under our feet, so we're always struggling to regain balance, to find our footing. It's hard to look forward when we must always be looking at the ground beneath us; we're more lurching than walking, stumbling to stay upright.

With constant adaptation, though, comes a remarkable resilience. When my original goals become unrealistic, I compromise. When those new goals become unrealistic, I compromise again. When my replacement-replacement goals become unrealistic, I get frustrated. And sad. But knowing that the range of what I'm capable of will shrink, I need to plan a life where my goals do not have to be slashed every year as my health declines. I can be creative with what I'm capable of as the limitations pile on. It's about perception—if careers are a means to an end (in my case, helping people and feeling challenged while making money to support myself), there have to be ways to get there that don't require a strict schedule, hard physical conditions, or sixty-hour workweeks.

Being frustrated and angry that something was taken from you hurts creativity, the very same creativity that could help you reinvent your possibilities and achieve your ends. Understanding this trap is important—knowledge is power.

So yes, CF does do a lot of taking. It's a complex, unpredictable, irreversible, progressive, painful, suffocating, choking weed of a disease and it's okay to hate it.

At the same time, it does give. It's given me the creativity to reimagine my life, a skill I wouldn't have needed to develop if everything had been easy and nothing was impossible.

It's given me a community of men and women who astound me every day with the strength and endurance they use to ride through daily challenges and life-or-death struggles. We all know this disease delivers both in big doses.

It's given me a way to cut to the chase in my friendships and relationships. Can you hang? Is that same person who's there when I'm laughing and partying going to be there when I'm sick or sedated? It's given me a resounding understanding of the value of a good friend, and my incredible luck in having so many.

It's given me the chance to look normal; not all diseases are so forgiving. It's a blessing and a curse not to look sick—a curse when I need accommodations but aren't given them because of the perception that I'm too healthy—but mostly, it's a blessing. I am not branded by illness on a daily basis. If I choose to disclose, it's just that: a choice.

It's given me a second home in the hospitals where I've had some of the best and worst moments of my life. I graduated college, officially (finished my last final), in the hospital. I've spent birthdays and holidays in the hospital. I've had panic attacks in the hospital. I've struggled to breathe in the hospital. I've forged powerful relationships with doctors, nurses, and ancillary support teams in the hospital. I've been grateful for the care I've gotten in the hospital. I've seen the strength of my family tested in the hospital. I've seen my own strength tested in the hospital.

It's given me the mountain that's been waiting for me all my life. The mountain we're all climbing, every day. It looks different for everyone, but we all have our own struggles, every person I see on the street. I have to remind myself not to envy those whose lives look normal, because their mountains do exist, even if they're less obvious than mine.

It's given me empathy, and gratitude, and courage, and humor, and heartache, and happiness.

All that giving balances all that taking and, in the end, I'm still here, in my second home in the hospital, having some of my best and worst moments, feeling at times like I'm going nowhere but knowing that, in reality, like Dr. Seuss told me I would, I'm getting on my way.

SALT IN MY SOUL

PART ONE

Mallory was always the tallest, smartest, most athletic girl in the grade—even at five years old. We'd chase boys around the playground and she'd run faster than all of them. They all had crushes on her. Mal was every teacher's favorite student, and every kid wanted to be her friend. She was the friend whose advice everyone wanted: she coached you when to text or not text the boy you liked, how to say the right things to convince your parents to let you go to that party, and gave you the best hug when you needed it most. Mal was the girl who missed forty days of the school semester and still got the highest grade in the class. She was the girl who laughed so hard she snorted, which made her laugh even harder. She was the prom queen— and would hate that I wrote that.

—TALIA STONE

2008

5/1/08—(Age 15)

About me: I could go every day to the beach and never get sick of it. I am obsessed with salt water going up my nose and seeing fish swim around my feet. I live for the grimy feeling of sand in my scalp. When I cry, the only thing I want to do is jump in the ocean.

I like change. It's exciting. Most people are afraid of it, but I embrace it. I hate when people say to each other, "You're changing," as if it's a bad thing. I think that at such a young age it's impossible to know entirely who you are and who you want to be.

I miss a lot of school.

I like lists. Actually, I like crossing things off lists. It makes me feel accomplished.

I love my family. My immediate family (Mom, Pidge = Dad, Bridge = Micah, Maria = our housekeeper who I love like family, and my animals) is really amazing. We have a good dynamic; all of us are so different. I think I'm the most normal one.

I'm deathly afraid of death.

I'm going on a permanent diet starting today. I'm going to eat less . . . and absolutely no sugar.

I probably won't be able to follow the zero sugar thing but I'm going to try really, really hard. And the only protein I'm going to eat is fish. I just want to be skinny and feel good internally and good about my body and right now I'm none of those things. I used to be considered thin and now I'm not, and that really bothers me. Because it's extremely hard to go from being thin to being "buff." Also, the doctors always say that I'll probably get diabetes, but if I eat no sugar then maybe not, because I already eat less sugar and I've lowered my blood sugar number from 159 to 85. I pretty much reversed inevitable diabetes! I'm ecstatic about it since I don't need any more conditions to worry about in addition to what I already have.

I read a lot. I read because the vast wholeness of existence (the immeasurable, multifaceted beauty of what it means to be human) cannot be perceived through one life.

I read because there are a lot of things I can't do. I'll never be like the characters of *On the Road,* picking up and hitchhiking across the country on a whim, living off cheap liquor store commodities and sleeping wherever there's no law against lying down. But through the eyes of the character Sal I got to see the beauty of spontaneity and the sheer emptiness of wandering forever and never setting down roots.

I read because I want to see things in my head that aren't actually there; I want to know about emotions that I've never felt before so that maybe if I do feel them they'll be recognizable. I want to relate to characters that may be a million miles away but still share so much with me because we're united by the human condition.

I read because we race through the millions of events in our lives, taking note only of the "milestones," but each of these events, even insignificant ones like biking by a tree as a leaf falls, can take on a distinct meaning when a writer observes its poignancy. A writer gets to choose which of these events are important, which to put in his writing, and which are mundane; but to do so, he has to *think* about all of these seemingly meaningless settings and backgrounds and occurrences on a deeper level than we ever do in our lives.

I like to write, but outside of school I've never had any reason to. There is so much out in the world to see and think about. I used to keep all my thoughts in my head, but eventually there was simply too much to keep it all straight, which is why I started this journal.

I've always wanted to be able to look back at some tangible body of writing and see the evolution of my outlook, how my beliefs and feelings and thoughts have changed over time in response to my life experiences. The records we leave behind of our lives as we grow older and pass away have always fascinated me; some people make scrapbooks, some people write novels, and some people document their lives through their actions. I have an interest not only in legacy, but also memory . . . in how, as time goes on, what was once vivid, real, *present,* becomes slippery and vague and trickles away like water cupped in your hands. I want to be able to look back and see not my actions, not my accomplishments, not my appearance, but the changes in my worldview and perspective.

My guess is the writing I do will grow to become a collection of ramblings and opinions about the food industry, nutrition, and agriculture; religion, philosophy, and animal rights; nature photography and environmentalism; recipes, good songs, quotes; and perhaps a bit of a cystic fibrosis lifestyle guide. Sometimes I just write about my day. No agenda, just thoughts from a girl who loves wildlife, the outdoors, swimming, hiking, surfing, volleyball, photography, literature, writing, new friends, old friends, sunrises and sunsets, friendly strangers, traveling, great music (country, folk, rock, reggae, and world music), barbecues, strong coffee, food, the Hawaiian Islands, happy memories, and every single day I get to live healthy.

I've grown up in a household that's all about food. My mom markets daily, sometimes hitting the produce market in the morning for fresh fruit and vegetables and then a different market just because it has this coffee she is obsessed with, and then a supermarket for the staples. I eat a hot breakfast every morning, have a healthy lunch packed for me, and come home each night to dinner on the table. When my friends and I are looking for a place to hang out before or after water polo or volleyball practice, we come to my house, knowing something fresh will be coming out of the oven.

But my mom isn't the only one in the household whose cooking is impressive. My dad makes a mean Chicken Marbella, meticulously marinating and chopping and spicing to ensure maximum flavor. While my mom uses whatever is in the house—which could be any random hodgepodge of ingredients—to miraculously create a meal from it *fast,* my dad is more of the gourmet, take-your-time kind of chef. My mom cooks every day, my dad cooks a few times a year.

They have between fourteen and twenty-two over for dinner every Sunday night, a tradition they started to feed my coach. It's always fun.

5/6/08
Letter to my teacher:

> You asked me to tell you why I haven't been in class. I was growing four types of infection in my lungs and the options were to be hospitalized for another round of IV antibiotics or to do extra treatments at home. I decided on the latter, which means adding one in the middle of the day (during your class). That's also why I wasn't in STAR testing.* You said you didn't understand how I could choose to go to a

---

* STAR refers to California's Standardized Testing and Reporting program.

swim meet instead of your class. My doctors drilled in me that health comes first, athletics second, school third. That might contradict your thinking, but swimming is extremely important in keeping me healthy and skipping it for a quiz is not an option. I hope you understand why what you said offended me because I care about doing well in your class, and missing school is not my choice but a necessary evil. I understand that you were annoyed about so many students wanting to make up tests on their own time, and I'm sorry to have to ask. I will see you tomorrow for the quiz.

5/19/08

I'm going to help my mom raise money for the Cystic Fibrosis Foundation!! Maybe my friends will, too. . . .

10/9/08

Frustrated about volleyball. As a team, we're letting negative expectations and thoughts affect the way we play. Mentally, we're not strong enough to disregard our doubts, fears, or frustrations. For a while now, we've been losing very close matches, and it's not due to lack of skills. It's because we get scared that we will lose, and this fear causes us to lose. It's hard to cast away fear.

What we need is to replace our desire to be perfect with a desire to do everything to the best of our abilities. Ball control is important—but we get so wrapped up in the need to be perfect that we end up making more mistakes because we get frustrated. When we mess up, we should become more determined, but instead when we mess up, we get scared that we aren't capable of doing better and begin to doubt our abilities.

Individually, it's hard to keep yourself focused and determined when you are pissed off or frustrated, which is why it's the responsibility of the team as a whole to bring everyone's attitudes up and make everyone more determined to work as a team to get each point. Negativity is contagious, and if we don't get rid of it, our season will continue to be plagued by losses.

We should only be satisfied with losing if we've given it our all.

10/23/08

What I wrote to the guy from Santa Monica High who was mean about Micah at their last water polo game:

Micah is my brother and I can vouch that he takes no steroids or creatine or whatever you accuse him of doing. He is an amazing athlete with an incredible work ethic. He works so hard to help his team win. That's right. You guys can wallow in your defeat and know that the Beverly Hills High School water polo team rocks. I'm good friends with many of the players and Coach Bowie is almost like my dad. You know that athletic ability comes AFTER good sportsmanship and mental toughness, right? If you ever want to beat Beverly you better improve your bad attitudes and accept that we're BETTER, FASTER, STRONGER, and we work harder. FYI, every single boy on the Beverly Hills water polo team is kinder, more athletic, funnier, and a better overall man than anyone on your team.

10/28/08

Today was a hard loss to deal with. Recently I haven't been playing as well as I know I can. No one has been. We all want to win; we just don't know how to accomplish it. I wish everyone knew how good we could be.

Last year during school season, I never thought I would play back row in my career; I didn't think it was one of my strengths, and so it never occurred to me I would come to care so much about it. In club volleyball I was exposed to a whole different mentality: defense and serve/receive make or break games. That was when I started to have a passion for back row, and once I got a taste of what it was like for a team to depend on me in back row (earlier this season), I knew that it would always have more meaning for me than hitting. I understand more now how much of volleyball is mental.

11/10/08*

Thin green blades beneath my bare feet poke, caress and comfort,
As unseen, unknown blades stab me from the inside out
In the delicate labyrinth, the network of frail scarred tubes
That is at once sustaining me and failing me.
Red splatters across the green,
The hated flag of sickness soiling nature,
Tarnishing my one escape.

I stand, walk, cough, sit, spew, swallow, stand again.
Green stretches before me, the lawn steep, security far.
I drop my books . . . cough.
Drop my backpack, cover my mouth . . .
Cough, spew, swallow, cough, spew, swallow.
Standing again, a deep breath incomplete, cough, spew.

---

* Mallory wrote this poem at Cedars-Sinai Medical Center, Los Angeles, during one of the earliest of her sixty-seven hospitalizations. Mallory was admitted for a "tune-up," what the CF community calls an inpatient stay to treat a CF exacerbation, a term coined to make it easier for kids to understand. We say, you take your car in for a tune-up and kids with CF need tune-ups, too. The primary purpose is to get a PICC line (peripherally inserted central catheter), so that intravenous antibiotics can be administered. Mallory was admitted for lung function decline and intermittent fevers.

The red is runny like water but sticky like glue.
In between gagging, coughing, spewing:
"Call . . . my . . . mom."
More coughs, the red still spews forth.
My lungs are wet
with the runny, sticky red.

Ambulance men say, "You're not sick;
you look great."
Mom yells. Grandma yells. Doctor yells.
I don't get sirens. I'm "not sick."
I "look great."
But my lungs are wet
With the red, runny and sticky.
Cough.

Emergency Room.
White walls, white sheets, white doctors
Make the red redder.
"How much?"
"No idea."
"How much?"
"No idea."
"How much?"
THIS FUCKING MUCH.

8:00 a.m. Vitals. Breakfast
Lots of eggs, whole milk.
Isolation. Mask and gloves.
Doctor A: "Three weeks here."
Doctor B: "Three days here."

Routine disagreements, I'm not to worry.
"This is an art, not a science. We learn as we go."
"You're not sick," says Nurse.
"She's very sick," says Mom.
To pass the time, I sit.
I stare at the walls.

12:00 p.m. Vitals. Lunch
Broccoli, beef stew.
Isolation. Mask and gloves.
Put it on when you come in;
Throw it away when you leave.
Doctors. Nurse. Respiratory therapist.
Fellow. Physician. Cleaning.
Put it on when you come in;
Throw it away when you leave.
To pass the time, I sit.
I stare at the walls.
Visitors, friends!
I sit, baring teeth,
Almost a smile but not quite.
"How ya feelin'?"
"Fine."

5:00 p.m. Vitals. Dinner
Beans, whole milk, fries.
Swollen arms, stiff knees, puffy eyes, dry skin.
The parade of people comes and goes.
Phone calls try to distract me.
"How ya feelin'?"
"Fine."
To pass the time, I sit.

I stare at the walls.
I lie in bed
All day, all night
But get no rest.

Sunday morning:
"You may leave," says Doctor A.
"Is she OK now?" says Mom.
Some gibberish. I guess.
Ripping tape,
Removing tubes,
Signing forms,
Baring teeth.
Time to leave please, to pursue freedom.
Mom let's leave please.
"My, you're tall," says Nurse.
"Yes."
She hadn't seen me stand.
I say good-bye,
To those who will stay.

Outside:
Air, sunshine and salt,
Nature, my escape.
A deep breath . . .
Freedom!
Love this.
Drowning in the flood of relief,
Strangled by my fleeting fortune.
Gone from that place,
Free at last!
Except not.

Never free of these unseen blades, which stab me from the
inside out
In the delicate labyrinth, the network of frail scarred tubes
That is at once sustaining me and failing me.

2009

9/5/09

My earliest wants were immediate, visceral, primal: Food! Water!
Mommy, I'm tired. Mommy, my head hurts. I want to play; can
we go to the park?

A blink later, the memories begin to materialize like figures
approaching in the dark. Still far away, I can just begin to make
out the shaded features of this person, Memory. I vaguely recall
postponing bedtime for string cheese, telling Dad everything
hurts ("Even your toenails?" "Yes, even my toenails!"), fearing the
creaks and sighs of the floorboards of our century-old house.
When I dreamed of Biter the dinosaur, I woke up screaming;
now, as a teenager with occasional paranoid tendencies, I realize
that my child-self-distorted-hours spent watching *Barney* and *The
Land Before Time* had morphed into the nightmares that plagued
me throughout childhood. One night, we laid food out for Biter
outside the door to my room: bread in a bowl, saturated with
milk, covered in chocolate chips and sprinkles, and made "appe-
tizing" with green food coloring fit for your average neighborhood T-Rex. That night, Biter showed up in my dreams yet
again—but he asked to be friends. For years after that, we galli-
vanted each night through tangled jungles and wooded nirvana.

My dad and I continued to put food out—to befriend the monsters before they had a chance to come get me.

At school, I had to go to the nurse's office at recess and lunch to get the pills I take every time I eat. In fourth grade, Ms. Lightner would hand me a Scandishake, a 600-calorie milkshake for weight gain, in the middle of class. I dawdled on the drinking, despite knowing that she would check to make sure I sucked every last drop. I snuck M&M's with no pills sometimes, aware of the stomachache I would get later, but itching to exercise some childish autonomy. My mom packed me a hot lunch for school every day: a thermos filled with mashed potatoes, brisket and gravy, or pasta Bolognese cooked with added butter. I just wanted the pita–Nutella sandwiches my friends had.

My tactics to postpone bedtime transformed in middle school from faking hunger to "Just one more paragraph!" as I read another chapter. Books seemed to stack themselves up in my room, calling me to read them. I lost myself in those worlds and will never forget the first time a book made me cry. At the end of *Clan of the Cave Bear,* when Ayla is banished from the Neanderthals and sets off alone to find her own kind, I bawled as if I were Ayla and I had been kicked out of my home. I pondered how beautiful the name Ayla is, and decided to name my future daughter Ayla. Then I remembered Elsa, the lioness from *Born Free,* and was temporarily conflicted about which name I would use for my own progeny.

Sometimes, if I went to bed too late, my mom wouldn't wake me up for school the next day. Her number-one concern was that I get enough sleep, classes be damned. I would finally awake on my own at 10:30 or 11:00, look at the clock, and start yelling about the math or spelling test I had missed. She always called the school; they were always fine with it. But I was not. I wanted to be there alongside everyone else, not in my bed sleeping the day away, receiving special treatment for a disease that hardly affected me at that point.

By eighth grade, I was tall and gangly. The dreaded awkward phase was under way, with my daily uniform of athletic shorts, baggy T-shirts, and braces. I wanted my first crushes not to be six inches shorter than me. In the annual school pageants, I wanted to be in the front row with my petite best friends. Everything was organized by height, so anytime we were onstage, I was in the far right corner of the last row, seated next to the next tallest person in the grade, a boy who sweetly and jokingly called me "Too Tall." I still played basketball at that age, so I preferred the nickname Too Tall to my other one: "Shaquille O'Neal."

My mom's friends would say "She's going to be a heartbreaker, that one." I would smile and, in my head, think how ridiculous that was—I would never be breaking hearts.

9/7/09

Can't believe it's my senior year of high school. I'm not ready to move out and start my life. I don't feel like an adult, I don't wanna act like an adult. Adult life seems so structured and tame. Adults have so many responsibilities, they lose their sense of humor. It just seems like everything goes downhill from the time you're twenty-five, and especially once you get married. Because once you're married, you have no freedom, no independence, no privacy, no time for friends. Maybe I just think this because I don't know anyone I would ever want to marry.

I want to make the most out of my senior year because after that, either everyone will go to college and I'll go too, or I'll take a year off, but either way everyone will separate and it will feel like I didn't get enough time in high school. Or maybe after this year I'll be ready to leave. I'm just not ready now. I like living at home, having friends I've known forever, and don't know how I'm going to handle not having anyone I know around me. Starting all over seems enormously difficult. I think that's why I haven't been able to make a college list. Because I can't picture myself at any school . . . I just keep picturing myself in high school forever. It's gone by so fast and college will go by even faster.

10/3/09

I haven't written in sooo long.

Time to think about college apps—Stanford? Or somewhere with parties? But do I even wanna party? Who do I wanna be when I grow up? The one who partied all through college or the intellectual one who never wanted to party? If I'm at a party and I always wanna drink = bad. I don't necessarily want that, maybe I just want something low-key . . . maybe I'm not fun. . . .

On another random note . . . am I an intellectually interested person? Am I a fun-loving, outgoing person? Or do I lean more toward quiet and reserved? I don't even know who I am. None of these qualities consistently describes me. I have no clue who I am. What do I enjoy? Sometimes I just enjoy being in my bed and eating, which is why I do it so much and why I hate my body so much because I just eat and eat and eat.

Maybe this is why it's so hard for me to write a college essay, because you have to write about who you are and I have no idea who I am. I can't pick a college because I have no idea who I am. The qualities that people always say I have—that I'm persevering, positive, determined—I don't feel like I'm any of those things. I happen to have a disease and do what the doctors tell me to do so that I don't die. I don't call that persevering. What choice do I have? It's not noble, like I sacrificed myself and took this on and am bearing the burden so well. I just happened to get unlucky and I'm still alive, so people think I "persevere." Positive? I guess I seem positive at times. But sometimes I feel like I'm a negative person. Not just about having a disease, but about everything. My hope is that I can learn to always be a nice, friendly, positive person, and lose the negativity.

Other times I'm happy, and it's the stupidest, simplest little things that put me in the best mood. When you can drive with the top down, listening to an amazing song, and just be happy, then you must be a person capable of happiness. What kinds of things make me happy? Daytime, but not when it's too hot. Driving and listening to country music, when I'm not in a rush and there's no traffic. Laughing really hard. A really good, healthy meal that doesn't make me extremely full. Actually, eating healthy in general because then I feel like I have some willpower and control.

As opposed to today . . . I ate two breakfasts, two lunches, dinner, and dessert. Ew. Carbs and fat. When I have absolutely no control over what I eat it's repulsive.

I need some resolutions. I would love it if I could remain a tolerant person. I've always prided myself on not being racist or elitist or discriminatory, but I really don't know what I am anymore. I'm second-guessing everything about myself right now.

10/4/09

My treatments are now close to an hour and a half and I can never bring myself to do homework during them so it's annoying and feels like I'm wasting time. Like right now, it's 11:30 on a Sunday night and I should be sleeping for school tomorrow, but I've been doing treatment since 10:00 and am not even done.*

---

* Mallory's treatments changed over time. She started with two treatments a day consisting of inhaled meds, between twenty-five and sixty pills a day, and chest percussion therapy. As she got sicker and her lung function declined, there were longer and more frequent treatments required and a layering on of IV antibiotics.

10/14/09

I don't know what I'm doing, all my work is building up, I feel like I've done nothing, I still have a million college essays, and when I have a ton of stuff to do (like tonight) I sit here instead and write about it in this journal, which is not productive. But I think it helps me mentally.

While I was doing treatment tonight, my parents came in and started talking about time management and staying healthy . . . blah, blah, blah. And they told me that I don't work hard in treatment, which made me SO mad.

People always say, "When you're stressed just remember that none of this will matter." But it will matter. If I am too tired to do a good treatment, like I have been for the past week or two, then the mucus builds up and affects me in every other aspect of my life.

I am so sick and tired of reading and tests and quizzes and scores. I want to be able to say one night, I'm a little tired so I'm gonna take it easy and watch a movie. Right now every single minute of every day is scheduled, and I hate that. And I'm always late. It's like a sign of my disorganization and constant stress that I can't get up in time to get to school on time. I forget things, I lose stuff, every room that I enter is a mess.

10/18/09

I think I'm really afraid of change and the future and I hold on to the past. Every time something happens I feel the need to write about it. I always want to have photos and I'm hugely afraid that Facebook could crash and all my pictures could be lost. I don't ever want to forget anything, and it scares me that things from as recent as freshman and sophomore years of high school and sometimes even junior year are starting to blur in my memory. Even the summer before junior year is pretty vague. I regret not writing more. Because for some reason I want to remember every little detail. Is that normal?

I don't want to forget what my favorite song is (though it constantly changes), or my favorite band (Counting Crows), or what books I like, or how I feel about my classes, or what school is like in general, or what I do on weekends and who I hang out with, and what is going on with my family, and who I am close with and who I'm not, and basically all the stuff that goes on. I want to remember all my trips, all my hospitalizations/IV antibiotics, all my adventures with my friends, all the times that are not memorable but just make me happy because they're simple, normal life moments that are nice.

I know that college will be amazing, but I haven't had enough of what my life is now. And a lot of it I don't even remember. Like Camp Hess Kramer: I remember it was amazing, but it's a distant memory. And I didn't write about it at all, so as distant as the memory is now, I probably won't even remember that I went there in twenty years. Junior and senior years are such a short part of my life, a year and a half of the seventeen years that I've lived, and I want to remember more. Or I want to start over and live it over again or go back a few years. I'm just not ready to give it up yet, but my friends seem to be ready to be done. Moving out? I'm a CHILD. It's a joke to think that I could live on my own. I sit in my bed that is ten feet from the kitchen and ask my mom to bring me green beans. I ask my mom to email my teachers when I get too sick to finish an assignment on time (or when I miss too much school) and I ask my dad for tutoring constantly. I'm not ready to be done with days like yesterday, when my dad and Micah and I went to Best Buy to get some batteries.

And Maria! Just sitting in the kitchen in the morning, when she asks me what I want for breakfast and I try to be as nice as possible despite my grouchy morning self. I'm gonna miss her so much in college! I just wish my family could come with me to college.

10/18/09

I completely forgot to write about my birthday! I hung out with Marissa and Talia and we were gonna go out and do something but it was freezing outside and none of us could drive each other so we ended up putting on pajamas and just chilling at my house. Then at night I went over to Jason's for dinner and Eileen made a really nice dinner for our families and a few friends.

10/22/09

I'm freaking out because I only have one weekend to finish the entire Stanford application. It's going to be ridiculously stressful next weekend. I'm applying early even though I didn't initially want to go—it didn't seem fun at all. But Ann* told my mom I should apply there because she said it's the perfect school for me. I've come to understand that Stanford attracts the brightest minds, the most well-rounded students and stellar athletes, and offers an impressive array of programs. But the hospital is also a huge draw. My CF protocol calls for monthly visits to monitor my lung function and to prevent progression of the disease, so it would make life much easier to be on a campus with such an amazing CF center. My recurring and frequent episodes of hemoptysis** will likely require embolization*** and there's a doctor at Stanford Hospital who is widely considered to be one of the top specialists in this field.

* a family friend who works as a college admissions advisor
** the coughing up of blood or blood-stained mucus from the bronchi, larynx, trachea, or lungs
*** a procedure to reduce or cut off the supply of blood that's performed by an interventional radiologist

Stanford also has an amazing culture—Division I sports to watch, club sports to participate in, mild weather, and a general culture of athletic activities such as bike riding, running, and hiking.

Because of my disease I'm not able to travel, which might be why studying foreign cultures is so appealing. The interdisciplinary major in the School of Humanities and Sciences would allow me to study Spanish works of art, literature, philosophy, and current issues that plague Latin American society.

12/12/09

I GOT INTO STANFORD!!!!!!!! I can't believe it. I'm so happy!!! The hard work that I've done my ENTIRE LIFE has paid off. I no longer have to have perfect grades. I got into one of the best schools in the country . . . in the world! What was it about me that made them accept me?? I'm just in shock. And I'm really proud and really relieved and really happy.

I was at my water polo tournament when I found out. I was standing there in my parka freezing my butt off when I got a call from Solange who said that Stanford had sent emails about their decisions and that she got deferred and she said to check and call her back.

I was trying to get the Internet on my BlackBerry and it was taking soooooo long to connect, but finally it did and I opened it and read: "Congratulations! On behalf of the Office of Undergraduate Admissions, it is my pleasure to offer you admission to Stanford's Class of 2014." My jaw just dropped and I started jumping and I screamed and I told my mom and then my whole team freaked out.

My mom looked SO happy for me—a surprise given that I know she wanted me to go to UCLA. But she knew my dad thought it was the right place for me and maybe she got caught up in the emotion of the moment. That or she's a good actress.

I don't even remember how or who I told but somehow everyone found out. And everyone started writing on my [Facebook] wall and calling me and texting me to say congratulations, and it was a pretty amazing feeling. It was sweet, and everyone was saying how much I deserved it.

2010

4/6/10

Before starting seventh grade, I came home from four weeks at camp having lost ten pounds from my already scrawny frame, as well as 30 percent of my lung function. On the second day of school I was admitted for my first hospitalization; before that, my lung function had never dipped below the 90s. My parents were terrified, but to me, even though I started out crazy upset, it was sort of an adventure. I got to spend way more time with friends than I normally did, because they came and brought me food and flowers and papered the walls with photos and cards. And I could read to my heart's desire, something I never had time for with school.

During that hospital stay, we received bad news, a test result that would change the course of my life: my lungs were colonized with the deadliest strain of the deadliest bacteria known to CF lungs, *B. cenocepacia*. My strain of *B. cepacia*, *cenocepacia*, is most associated with rapid clinical deterioration, high virulence, resistance to most antibiotics, and high post-transplant mortality. It doesn't start as a superbug but over time it morphs into one from

antibiotic resistance. I overheard Dr. Pornchai* telling my mom
that this was terrible news and that things would be very different
for me from then on. I didn't understand what all the fuss was
about, and the adults were happy to keep it that way. I actually felt
fine, and by then was ready to be done with this whole hospital
business and get back to school. As a seventh grader, esoteric
medical terms and distant notions of death meant very little to me.

Now, in the second semester of my senior year of high school, I
find myself in the intermediate ICU wing of UCLA's new medical center. I was admitted after my lung function and weight had
both steadily declined for two months, until both were no longer
acceptable. Despite the 2,000 calories of lipids being pumped into
my veins each day, in addition to the 3,000 calories I am forced to
eat, my weight loss continues; the *B. cepacia* infection is acting up,
causing pneumonia, and my body is in full-scale battle mode,
fighting it. Disease-fighting processes burn a lot of calories.

Outside of the hospital, my swim team friends are at the peak
of training intensity to prepare for league finals, and prom is coming. Stanford is sending me information about Admit Weekend,
graduation speaker auditions are being held, teachers have given
up thinking the seniors still care about their classes, and friends are
finally putting old grievances aside and making the most of their
last few months together. As the days wear on, I grow more
oxygen-dependent, experiencing pain with breathing, and am no
longer able to walk without help.

During my third week in this hospitalization, Talia came to
visit. She sat at the foot of my bed and we made conversation,

* The head CF doctor at Cedars-Sinai then, later the head CF doctor at UCLA

although I had to catch my breath after every few words. Two long tubes ran from the IV pole to my PICC line; one was filled with a milky white fluid, pure fat, and the other contained a clear but potent antibiotic. Both were delivered to my heart to be circulated throughout my body.

That day, a knock at my door announced the arrival of Dr. Pornchai for his daily rounds. He'd been my doctor since Dr. Bowman moved back east to start a new CF center. Dr. P was warm, with a shy demeanor, but he took an aggressive approach to his advanced lung disease medical practice; his knowledge and experience inspired confidence in all of his patients. But that day, he seemed hesitant, nervous. He asked Talia to leave; no doctor had ever asked a friend of mine to leave the room before. Already shivering from fever, my body began to tremble with agitation. What was he about to tell me? Whatever the bad news was, it had to mean my health was not turning around. My mom closed the door. I could see the fear in her eyes.

"Mallory, your weight has dropped again today, to 136, and your white blood count has climbed to 19,000. The lipids are not working," he said, in his low voice I'd grown to love. "The results of the sensitivity analysis on your sputum will not be ready for a few days, but you are not responding to the current trio of antibiotics. I'm very concerned. Your case is extremely complicated and I do not have enough experience with *B. cepacia* to know where to go from here. I have contacted some top hospitals to see what other options we have."

His voice broke on "complicated." In all my time as his patient, I had never seen him look afraid, let alone invoke the help of another center. Doctors do not generally show emotion to their patients, but Dr. Pornchai had watched me grow up. More than that, he had made my growing up possible. And I loved him. In that moment, his eyes began to water. He understood mortality far better than I, having seen firsthand how *B. cepacia* can reside in stable coexistence in the lungs for years and then randomly, rapidly, turn into a deadly killer.

Dr. Pornchai performed a bronchoscopy, a procedure that suctions mucus from the lungs and provides a specimen that can be sent out for a more accurate culture. To remove as much mucus as possible in order to help combat the pneumonia, he directed the scope deeper than he normally would have, into the fragile, thin airways at the base of my lungs. A tiny puncture was all it would take for the *cepacia* to leak into my blood.

I woke up from the bronchoscopy in a disoriented and feverish sepsis. Four nurses held me down on the bed as my entire body convulsed violently and erratically, while my fever quickly climbed from 103 to 104, then to 105, up to 106. More nurses arrived to cover my face and limbs with ice packs. I remember the pain, confusion, and disorientation, the sea of faces towering over me trying to soothe me, the nausea, the feeling of bathing in fire, and the terror of feeling like I was sitting off to the side, watching my body thrash and writhe without having any ability to stop it. My mom was terrified.

This was the first time CF shook me by the shoulders and made me look it in the eye to see it for what it really was. There was no more sheltering. *B. cepacia,* a term that once had little impact on me, was now something that weighed on me daily. I learned that my strain can cause cepacia syndrome, which is when the bacteria spread throughout the body and cause death within a few weeks. I learned that my strain is a contraindication for lung transplant because only about a third of patients with *cenocepacia* survive to the five-year post-transplant marker, and many die from reinfection within a few months of transplant. I learned that my strain is not something to mess around with.

This hospitalization makes my reality seem sharper and more

vicious. Every decision at this point seems significant, every complication more ominous, and every day more precious.

4/26/10

So I'm out of the hospital and I went to school today! This last
weekend was Admit Weekend at Stanford, which was SO fun.
Thursday I got out of the hospital in the morning (wasn't clinically ready to be discharged but they thought it was important
for my psychological health to get to go). Went to lunch with
Grandma at Cabbage Patch, then home to pack, caught a 5:15
flight arriving in San Jose at 6:30 and to Uncle Danny's at 7:30.
I went to campus at 8:00 and joined a group of profros (prospec-
tive freshmen). Then we saw a group of twenty people going
into one of the dorms so we followed them. There was definitely a wide mix of people but they were all nice and it wasn't
awkward, it was fun. Then my parents came to get me because
I had to do treatment.

Both nights I had to leave campus by 10:00 or 10:30 because
of treatment, which is kind of annoying, but with two hours of
treatment keeping me up late I would have slept the whole next
day away. We stayed at Danny's, which was good because it would
have been insanely overwhelming and unsanitary and impossible
for me to stay in the dorms with IVs and treatment. Friday I woke
up, did treatment, drove to campus to check in, then went to the
activities fair. There were a million clubs and activities to choose
from and so many people, and it was warm and beautiful out. I
might try out for everything and see who wants me and what I
like the best.

Before this weekend I wanted to go to UCLA and I could
envision myself eating in the dorms, and swimming in the rec
center, and going to class and walking around campus and going
to parties at frats. But I realize that the only reason I envisioned

myself there so much more than Stanford was because I'd never seen that side of Stanford. I'd only known about how amazing it is academically, which is obviously good but which isn't the most important thing to me (I want balance). But besides the fact that it's an amazingly prestigious name, it's beautiful and looks like camp, and it also has a lot of convenience factors that make it feasible for me to go to school there. UVA was the school I initially wanted and loved when I visited. But it just wasn't realistic for me to even consider it because it doesn't have a good CF center (or any CF center at all, actually), it's across the country, there's no family nearby to help me if I needed anything, it's in a small town, I'd have no car, and it's cold.

At Stanford, the weather is perfect, it has an amazing CF center, I have connections to the doctors (Drs. Cornfield and Weill are both friends of Danny's), I have Danny's house about one mile from campus so if my roommate gets sick or I need to rest or clean my gear I can go there, I'm going to have a car with a handicap placard, and I'm only an hour's flight from home. It's as if someone created a school that has all the qualities that realistically I need in order for me to live away from home.

I went to my meeting with Teri Adams, who works for the Office of Accessible Education (OAE), which basically helps people with medical conditions and disabilities. She was pushing hard for me to get a single because she said most people with conditions like CF don't do well with roommates and she wanted to prevent any potential problems. I explained how important it was for me to have the experience of a roommate, to live with someone, to not be isolated, etc. I told her that some people have personality traits that make it difficult to live with them. My issues are the noise of the treatment, the space it takes up, the need to be clean and get to bed early. But I compensate by being really easygoing with everything else. I'm not the kind of person who wou

start drama with a roommate and I avoid conflict by finding reasonable solutions to problems. I think I'm an easier person to live
with than most despite all the medical stuff. She agreed that I
could have a roommate, and we decided that I would get a sink in
the room, and air-conditioning, and that I would take only two
classes fall quarter. It's better that way because I'm going to have
so much to get used to living on my own, which is going to take
up a ton of time. My daily regimen includes cleaning a million
different things like sinus rinse, eFlow,* nebulizers, etc., that my
mom used to do and I'm also going to be in a clinical trial, which
also takes time.

After dinner they broke us into groups for a scavenger hunt.
My group was Anna, Alex, Garrett, and a guy named Matt. It was
an interesting experience because Matt was blind and had a seeing
eye dog, so we went really slow. It was an eye-opening experience . . . because the rest of that day I was just so grateful that I
could *see*. He depended entirely on that dog and, although he
loved her, she wasn't perfect. At one point she did something
wrong and he walked into a bike and cut his leg, and whenever
there were curbs and street corners and stuff we would help him
because the dog wasn't doing a great job. It made me so sad but
he seemed to be a happy person despite his enormous limitations.
When we first got into our groups, he said, "Just so you know,
I'm probably not going to be very good at this," and it broke my
heart.

Walking around the campus, I realized how much of my happiness is based on seeing beautiful things in my environment, and
that's a whole part of life that he just completely misses out on. It's
funny how my mom always gives me the "perspective" talk but I
never really thought it worked until now. I can't believe how de-

---

*the device used to inhale Cayston, another antibiotic

pressed I was to be on IVs (the round before spring break). So I had to miss swimming. So I missed a few weeks of school. Wow, big deal! This guy is blind, and somehow maintains an outwardly positive attitude.

Saturday morning I had breakfast in the dorm with a bunch of random profros. I sat with a group of kids from New York who were pretty cool, and then I left to go to the athletic involvement meeting to introduce profros to club sports, wilderness programs . . . all the different ways to get involved in athletics. Afterward I asked the guy who was in charge of the wilderness program about the SPOT program (summer pre-orientation trip) to see if I could go on one of the trips with my treatment. He said the wilderness ones wouldn't be possible because they're backpacking so there's no electricity, but the rock climbing and community service ones both have a base where you stay, so I could do those. And he was really cute! But I don't remember his name. My mom asked him to show us where the gym was, so he started walking with us and then my mom was like, "Oops, Mal, I gotta go meet Dad, so you guys go along and call me after." Haha, so typical, she just wanted to leave me alone with him. Wingmom!!!

The last few months have been such a whirlwind . . . I went from my first round of IVs, during which I was basically doing nothing and watching TV all the time, to getting off and swimming in invitationals, then straight to Hawaii—amazing as always!! Then the day after I got home from Hawaii I went to the hospital, then the day I got out of the hospital I went to Stanford Admit Weekend. Last night was the first time sleeping in my bed since before spring break, so my first time since March. It's now almost the end of April. And APs are in one week!! Wowww. I have been out of school for a very long time. Today was my debut back. But I only went to one full class (Gov) and ten minutes of Math.

4/28/10

I should write the whole Dillon/prom story in here! Rob (my water polo coach) came to visit my first week in the hospital and asked me who I wanted to go to prom with. Somehow he figured out that I wanted to go with Dillon, Kyle, or Brandon and said he was going to bring all three of them to the hospital in their Speedos so I could pick. I started picturing it being like *The Bachelorette,* so I told him that could not happen. Before he left he told me that he was going to bring Dillon over to visit.

The next day he texted my mom, saying, "I'm bringing Dillon to visit on Wednesday," and I froze, wondering how the hell he got him to agree to that. Dillon and I weren't friends outside of school, we didn't have each other's phone numbers, we had never hung out! I was wondering what Rob said to get him to come visit me in the hospital, by himself, with no one else from the team. So I asked Rob, and he said he told Dillon straight up about prom. And I kinda freaked out imagining this. Apparently Rob asked Dillon privately if he would want to go to prom, and Dillon asked with who, and Rob said Mallory, and he said yes. And Rob said he seems interested but nervous. Then on Wednesday Dillon came with Rob. It was awkward but really funny because he was there to talk about prom but we weren't talking about it. We went down to the cafeteria for dinner (Rob, Dillon, my mom, and me) and then we came back to the room and hung out there. Right before they were gonna leave, Rob said, "So, are we gonna make this official?" and we just sort of stared at each other. Finally Rob said, "Dillon, do you wanna go to prom with Mal?" and he said, "Yeah," and then, "Mal, do you wanna go to prom with Dillon?" and I said, "Yeah." It was like the minister at a wedding. And my mom was on the other side of the room pretending not to listen but I'm sure cracking up.

The next day my mom gets a text from Dillon. He was going

to come visit but she didn't tell me anything else. So then this afternoon I'm sitting in my hospital room alone (my mom left because I guess he asked her not to be there) and he walks in with flowers and his jacket zipped up all the way. He said Tamara told him about the tradition of asking in a cute way (which I wanted). He hands me the flowers, unzips the jacket, and his shirt underneath has written on it, "Is this cute enough?" in Sharpie. I was so happy he asked me in a "cute" way. And then he asked me to go to prom with him. He looked a little nervous and a little sheepish but it was SUCH a cute way to ask, he got an A+. Then he stayed for two hours and we had dinner in the cafeteria and hung out in my room. And it wasn't awkward at all, it was easy to talk to him when it was just the two of us. He seems to get shy around adults.

5/1/10

Today was Prom!! I woke up at 9:00. It was a beautiful day so I decided to work out! I ran to Beverly, did two sets of stairs, ran a total of one mile (but with breaks in between), and walked home. Then it was time to get ready!

Dillon arrived while I was trying to tape the edge of the dress to my skin so it wouldn't move around, so I quickly tossed all my medical stuff into my bag, then went into the living room to meet his mom and see him. He looked really good in his tux.

We took pictures in front of the house for a while, and it was kinda cute and kinda awkward, too. We left and went to Talia's pre-prom, and got there at 6:00, right when most people were arriving. It was amazing to see everyone all dressed up looking gorgeous.

Dillon was probably a little bit uncomfortable because he didn't know most of the people, but I introduced him to everyone. I quickly started IVs right before the limo came. It was really squished but still fun to be going to prom at the Sheraton at

Universal Studios. It was nicely decorated, way better than I expected. It was kind of club-like with lounge furniture and lighting
and stuff. So we go in, see everyone and talk to people for a while,
then we ate dinner, then everyone started dancing. It was fun
being with the whole grade and everything. Then around 10:00
they said they were gonna announce the prom court. So everyone
stopped dancing and they announced Rosie Kohn and Daniel
Bradbury as prom princess and prince, and then they said, "And
your prom queen is MALLORY SMITH." And I just stood there
stunned for about twenty seconds, not moving. And I thought I
was imagining it, I didn't even believe it until everyone started
looking right at me and all my friends were pushing me up to the
stage. So obviously I had no idea what to do with myself, I was
so shocked and awkward and confused! I got my tiara from Dr.
Tedford and went onstage but was behind a speaker so everyone
thought I was hiding. And then they announced that the prom
king was Kevin Hekmat!!

I was really happy because I think it's the first time I've ever
been voted anything by my peers. I've won things that teachers
and coaches have nominated me for, but this showed that my
friends/peers like and respect me and it was a good feeling. Especially because I didn't ask anyone to vote for me.

My jaw dropped when I heard it was me, and I think Dillon's
did, too. Afterward I was walking around the party and people
kept staring at me and saying, "Hi prom queen!" and one group
of people I've never met before pulled me into their picture. I was
really happy with my prom dress, which Jan, my mom's friend,
bought for me as a pity present when I was in the hospital. It was
SO extravagant and I loved it!

Crazy after-party story! After fifteen minutes of being at the
club on Robertson, saying hi to a few people, Natasha asked me

to come to the bathroom with her, so Dillon and I started following her and then I felt an itch in my throat and I felt him taking
my hand and leading me the opposite way. I was really confused
because I didn't understand why we weren't still following her to
the bathroom. And then my throat really started to burn, and my
lungs started searing a little bit, and my nose and eyes were water-
ing, and I coughed a little blood. I noticed that the whole party
was evacuating. Once outside, everyone was wondering what was
going on, and someone told me that a guy from a competing
after-prom party had set a tear gas bomb off. Which is really
fucked up, of course.

We were all sitting out there talking for a really really long
time, a bunch of drunk people staggering and some others smok-
ing. I was freezing. Eventually the security people started letting
people back in. But since I already felt the damage in my lungs, I
knew it would be stupid to go back in and risk more bleeding.
Natasha offered to stay out with me, but I told her to go back in,
and Dillon stayed out with me. Since the party was going strong
and it was freezing, we decided to walk down the street to Norms
Restaurant and get hot chocolate, which was really amazing since
it was sooo cold out. It was fun sitting in Norms but we weren't
laughing, we were both a little bit tired, but it was a really nice
night.

I'm home now, listening to "Kol Galgal" right now btw, by
Shotei Ha'nevuah . . . it's amazing. It kind of reminds me of *Lord
of the Flies* a little though, just like "Sullivan Street" reminds me of
Atonement.

5/15/10
Can't believe I was picked to give a speech at graduation!!! And
Jason gets to give one as Class President!!!

6/14/10

I'm graduating high school!! Beverly Hills High School has been my home for as long as I can remember. My life has revolved around sports, friends, schoolwork. I owe so much to this school. Sometimes I would complain that I didn't like it, or that I wished I went to a different school, but looking back on it, I can't imagine having a better high school experience.

What I'll remember most:

Driving to school in the morning with my wet hair and my hot tea, listening to music with the windows down, wind in my face, at 9:00 a.m.

Walking through the hallways, still sometimes getting lost even this year. Mr. Borsum's class—I've been in his class for three years now, and every year we do a little math and a lot of talking!

Morning practice. Yes, I will miss it!! Dragging myself out of bed at 5:20 in the morning on Monday, Wednesday, and Friday, having it still be dark, driving to school and jumping in the water, and having already exercised by the time it's 7:30 in the morning. I'm going to miss the physical aspect of it—it gets you in *such* good shape, and the social aspect of it—everyone having morning practice together, then afternoon, it really bonds you.

I'm going to miss living in my house with my family, waking up in the morning and seeing them, and seeing them before I go to bed. Having my dad sit with me while I do treatment and when I'm falling asleep because I don't like to be alone. I'm going to miss being in that stage of life where if you really need something, your parents can always make it happen. And this is the perfect stage of life, because they do so much for me, but I also have my independence and can do what I want. I'm going to miss Maria, and our half Spanish–half English conversations, and how she always tells me to clean my room but I never do.

I really hope I have fun in college, and that I make the most of everything. I hope my health doesn't worsen. Right now my lung function is 2.8 liters (down from my baseline of 3.4 liters) and they're thinking this might be a new baseline. I hope that with the clinical trial it goes back up, and I hope college life doesn't make me much worse.

I hope I'm as happy a person in four years as I am now. I'm really starting to appreciate what an amazing childhood I've had, and I'm both nervous and excited for the future. Senior year has been such a whirlwind . . . I'm starting to really get sad.

7/3/10

Pediatrics vs. adult care when I start Stanford? They tell me the main difference has to do with parental involvement and how they treat me in terms of who makes the decisions for my care. I've always been a pediatric patient but Stanford is telling me I get to make the choice. I just can't decide. They say peds is more nurturing, but I don't want to be treated like a child. I just don't know what's right for me. Since I'd have to be transferred to adult care if I get hospitalized (at eighteen they put you in the main hospital), why would I put off the inevitable? I may as well make the transition now.

7/10/10

Made the decision to go with the adult team and met them all on Wednesday, then did ten tests and started a clinical trial on Thursday for a new drug called ataluren.*

---

* Mallory had the Delta F 508 allele along with G 542 X. The first mutation was common. The second—referred to as a nonsense mutation—was not. There weren't any therapies in development that targeted nonsense mutations, so when we heard about a promising clinical trial (ataluren), we moved mountains to get her enrolled. Ataluren was supposed to work by causing the protein-making machinery of the cell to ignore the premature stop signal and continue reading the gene to produce the full-length

7/18/10

I've been too lazy and busy to write about what I'm doing, but I'm having a very good summer. I'm still working at Motive Entertainment doing PR for their movies, which I like. It makes me feel productive, gives me a reason to get up and out of the house, and it makes me feel independent. I've been going to the gym pretty much every day, doing yoga, spinning, and the elliptical. I need to start swimming again and I wanna go surfing, do real rock climbing, and paddling, and ocean swimming. I've barely been at the beach all summer, which is sad. I've just been soooo busy.

I can't even describe how I feel about going away. My days are so everyday, so normal, that I completely forget that I'm leaving so soon. My bathroom issues are DEFINITELY not resolved and it's nerve-wracking. I don't know how I'm going to deal with communal bathrooms in the dorms. If I can't figure it out, I predict that I'll just stop eating, especially if the food is unhealthy and makes me feel bad. That wouldn't be good because if my weight isn't stable, I can't be in the clinical trial. I have to go to Stanford three more times before school starts, once in July, once in August, once in the beginning of September. I'm on a twenty-eight-day schedule, which has to be exact, and I'm required to do the e-diary for ataluren every day, too.

---

protein. We hoped that ataluren would increase Mallory's levels of functional CFTR protein, improving mucus consistency and reducing the symptoms of CF.

Mal was finishing high school when the Phase 3 trial of the drug started. The trial was designed for patients to receive either ataluren or a placebo for forty-eight weeks at sites across North America, Europe, and Israel. Mallory enrolled at the Stanford site and started at the end of June 2010. We didn't know whether she got the study drug or the placebo for several years after, but during that first year she had zero hospitalizations, the first time in six years she wasn't admitted. She also easily gained twenty pounds after years of struggling to gain weight. Eventually we came to find out that she had been on the study drug.

No idea how to make the most out of a tiny dorm room so I don't go crazy from claustrophobia. I also have to get more comfortable riding a bike and being close to other people on bikes (now when I'm within ten feet of anyone on a bike, I get freaked out and start wobbling).

7/30/10

I got my ears and cartilage pierced!!! It really didn't hurt at all. People warned me it would hurt a lot but I think all my time with PICC lines and multiple IVs has made me capable of enduring a lot of pain.

And I've read so many books this summer: *By the River Piedra I Sat Down and Wept* by Paulo Coelho, *Cat's Cradle* by Kurt Vonnegut, *The White Tiger* by Aravind Adiga, *The Spirit Catches You and You Fall Down* by Anne Fadiman (for Stanford), and *Joe College* by Tom Perrotta.

8/15/10

On Saturday, I flew to Oregon with Becca, Willy, and Melanie—SO MUCH FUN! We went to be with Michelle and her family and went biking, toured everywhere (so many trees and meadows and beautiful skies and clean air), hung out by the pool, then went horseback riding. On Monday we went river rafting and it was AMAZING. We drove two hours to the river, rafted until 11:30, then stopped for lunch, but I couldn't eat because I had left my enzymes in the van. But I did do Cayston and took ataluren. We went back on the raft, going seven more miles down the river. Tuesday we went tubing all together—hilarious! Quite an arm workout. I was so sad to leave.

One great thing about the trip was that I discovered that

coffee makes me go to the bathroom! I would take Glycolax and nothing would happen, then have two cups of coffee and immediately go to the bathroom. I did all my treatments and all my own sterilizing of equipment and everything was totally fine. It made me much more confident about going to school.

PART TWO

I have never met an extraordinary student like Mallory in my twelve years of high school counseling. I wholeheartedly concur with her AP Calculus teacher, who commented, "When I fill out a college recommendation form, I take very seriously the column that states, 'One of the best of my career.'" Mallory will be one of only a very few that will have that box checked in my thirty-three-year career. This is true for both her academic skills and her personal qualities.

Mallory possesses emotional maturity, genuine altruism, moral integrity, academic genius, effective leadership, and outstanding citizenship that any prestigious institution would desire in a serious candidate. I cannot think of any other student who has made such a significant impact on the campus and in the community with genuine passion, vitality, and commitment. She has my highest recommendation for admission to Stanford University.

—DIANE HALE,
Beverly Hills High School College Counselor

9/15/10

Moved into my dorm yesterday and spent my first night here! I left L.A. on Sunday morning and drove up with Pidge while my mom and Micah flew up. No room in the car for them with all my stuff. We ate at an IHOP in the outskirts of Bakersfield where it was ninety-five degrees. We saw lots of cows and Central Valley scenery and when we got farther north, it was really beautiful with the lighting and the hills, especially when we were passing this huge reservoir. Sunday and Monday night we all stayed at Uncle Danny's, so I got to spend time with my cousins Sarah and Hannah and my Aunt Lissa. Monday I got up and ran around in Palo Alto, then went out to lunch with my family and Ali and her family at this amazing bakery called Mayfield, then I went with my mom and dad and Ali's family to get bikes!! I've never had my own bike before!! And then Tuesday, yesterday, I moved in!

I was shocked by how big my dorm room is! Way bigger than my room at home because they knocked down the wall between two mini-doubles and made it into a big triple. I didn't even know that Stanford had triples so it was definitely a surprise. I'm also soooo happy with whom they picked as my roommates. Sabrina and Adele are supportive of me and my special needs.

9/16/10

It's Thursday. I've been SO busy, I've barely had any time to sleep or do treatment. But it's been fun and new and exciting. I feel like I've been here for so long, and it's not weird to be here. I always thought it would feel weird to be away from home, but it definitely does not. I've barely even talked to friends from home because I'm so busy.

We had dinner and a dorm meeting where we went over rules and policies and did an icebreaker. I did ataluren and inhaled meds while the RA was talking, and this guy came over to me and asked what I was doing, why I was using a nebulizer, what my health condition was, whether it was mild, moderate, or severe, whether I would die soon, how I felt about it all, and whether I believed in God. We ended up in a thirty-minute conversation about God and religion vs. spirituality, and a lot of other stuff that is interesting to me.

People looked over and clearly wondered what was going on. It was a little off-putting at first, but I told myself to get used to people staring.

9/21/10

Monday I started classes!! One of my professors is Tobias Wolff!! He was SO interesting and funny. It's amazing to have such a famous professor! I'm excited for the class because of him, and because most of the teaching fellows seem smart and interesting, too. I did the first reading assignment and it was really good.

I had Physics at 3:00. That's going to be a hard class, I can tell. Actually, I'm supposed to be reading the first chapter right now, but I've been procrastinating all day! Because I'm scared it's going to be hard and that discourages me and I don't want to have to look around for another class, especially since this one fits so per-fectly in my schedule!

2011

1/1/11

I can't believe it's 2011! Where the hell did 2010 go? . . . And now it's New Year's Day. So many things to write about—fall quarter, Thanksgiving, winter break Maui trip with the family, winter quarter and being kinda depressed/self-image issues.

First, I did well on grades the first quarter yay! I got an A– in both Physics and Program in Writing and Rhetoric (PWR), and a B+ in Intro to Humanities. Next quarter I'm taking Poetic Justice (Russian Lit), Intro to Modern Europe, the Problem of God: From Aquinas to the New Atheism (an Introductory Seminar that I think is going to be really bomb), and Sleep and Dreams. I need to make sure I have time to take naps at least like three times a week, and that I have time to exercise every single day, and that I have time to do treatment, obviously.

If it's too much, I just don't know which one I would drop.

1/20/11

I'm in such a weird place mentally right now. Lately. I was before I went to Hawaii, near the end of last quarter and during the first week of winter break. And then I went into the sun, into my element, back to my roots with my family, in the place I love, and I felt like I knew myself again. I knew why I was here . . . why I actually *like* life. For the smell of the water and the feeling when you wake up and stretch your arms out in bed after a great night's sleep, and when your family's nearby and everyone's getting along, and a really great cup of coffee, and the breeze that whips your hair all around as you drive along in the sunshine. And the sunshine itself, the light and the warmth and the way it shines so much *potential* onto every day. And then when it's gone, that potential is just sucked away, it's a void, it's worry, it's anxiety, it's fatigue, and being sick of *everything*.

I'm not sure what's going on with me right now. I'm not sure if it's because I've got a cold and I'm a little sick so I'm more tired, and I had the huge stressful dilemma of not having a class schedule, being indecisive, not being confident in the fact that I would actually get through this quarter.

It feels like I'm at the mercy of the professors. I'm desperate, late, not on top of my shit, and already feeling like this quarter will be a failure when it's barely even started yet. I know I'm feeling this way because I'm behind, because there's so much work. I've come to realize *there will ALWAYS be work*. The work doesn't stop.

What about enjoyment? What about *joy*? Is there anything we do that's purely based on physical sensual *feeling*? What feels good, what tastes good, what sounds good, what we *want,* what we *feel like doing,* who we want to be, what we want to choose?

3/15/11

I was really nostalgic today and thinking about my entire past in little tidbits . . . about the randomest memories like Halloween last year with all my senior friends, and hanging out with Becca, Michelle, Erica, and Natasha, and going with my dad to Starbucks on a weekend and just sitting and talking. And having dinner with my whole family. And Maria. And Thanksgiving at Jason's, and when it would rain in L.A. and it would be so different and I'd come home and get in my sweats and drink tea and watch TV on the couch. And how when I was in middle school, I had these weird conceptions about high school (like that you could talk on the phone, or listen to music, or sleep during class and the teachers wouldn't care at all, because it was your responsibility whether or not you wanted to learn). And how I thought of college as being SO old, and SO far away, and then it just snuck up on me and here I am. How did I get here?

6/24/11

The decision to become vegetarian is something I've been thinking about since I was in elementary school but didn't do it then for two reasons: I wasn't allowed by my mom (she was worried I'd get sicker if I didn't have animal protein), and I didn't know enough to fight with her about it.

I've been learning a lot about the food industry in the United States since I took a class on food science and politics and learned about factory farming.

It reintroduced the issue of animal rights and the ethics of eating, which I hadn't thought about in a while. Now that I'm knowledgeable, I can't say that I care about the treatment of animals and humanity's impact on the environment while continuing to eat meat without feeling like a hypocrite.

I do know enough about nutrition to be able to get the protein that I need without eating meat, and I'm dedicated to making it a priority for now.

7/15/11

So much has happened since I last wrote. I'm in Hawaii!! I think I've been here nine days now. Quick recap of the end of the year: it was a blur saying goodbye to friends at school, trying to see friends in L.A., unpack and organize myself to be ready for Hawaii. Had to bring six weeks of medical supplies plus all my gear from L.A. to Palo Alto and then from Palo Alto to Hawaii.

It's amazing how I immediately started feeling better once I got here. I lost myself for a while during the year. But I changed in a lot of ways that were good (becoming more outgoing, more open, discovering what I want to do with my life, what my passions are, figuring out what kind of people I want to surround myself with, learning how to take care of myself, dealing with all the medical stuff, being independent, etc.). But also in some ways that were bad (coming to dread exercise, feeling bad about myself every time I would finish a workout). I lost all drive to exercise, didn't feel good about myself, had no control over what I was eating even when I knew it would make me feel sick.

That continued into L.A. but got a little better when I started doing yoga. It sucks because I'm so torn in two directions. I want to feel good and feel strong and healthy, and I feel that way when I'm in good swim shape and I do great swim workouts. But when I start doing that I notice myself bulking up and I realize that in some ways I feel better about myself when I'm more feminine and not so buff in the upper body and athletic and boy-looking. And then it's like I try to lose weight and eat healthy and all that (not a lot of weight, just like five pounds would be good)—but then if I start to feel sick in my lungs like I'm getting a bit of an infection, or I'm more irritated than usual in my coughing, then I'll eat because nutrition is therapeutic and fat fights infection.

So I'm constantly in battle. It's not even between appearances and health, because, if it was that simple, I like to believe I would just choose health and learn to love my body whatever it looks like. What makes it hard is that I actually *feel* better with my gastrointestinal system when I'm thinner and eating less (I don't get acid reflux, I don't get blockages, I'm not as fatigued, etc.), and I'm able to exercise more, which also makes me feel better. It's really not just about looks. But then again, when I'm bigger I feel better in my *lungs*. It's a huge trade-off.

I just LOVE being here because it's amazing how quickly I see the benefits. My mom was here Wednesday to Sunday of last week, and we went on Friday to the north shore. I rented a board and surfed for a while, then chilled, then swam in the ocean, then

went paddleboarding. And I felt SO good that night. I was bringing up so much mucus, feeling so clear, not waking up in the
middle of the night unable to breathe. The worst thing is when I
wake up in the morning and feel like I can't even stay standing long
enough to make breakfast, brush my teeth, get dressed. I don't
have that problem as much here. There's nothing comparable to
the ocean for me in terms of what makes me feel good.

9/20/11

First week of classes. I'm praying that I don't get hospitalized
this year. Last year was the first time in six years that I wasn't
admitted! I'm so happy to be back but finding it hard to study
and get work done. Having fun but worried about my lung
function. Splitting up treatments is not working, because I never
do the second half at night. Tomorrow I have clinic at 3:00.

9/27/11

My brain is really fuzzy right now because of the ridiculous
heat, so I can't even remember what happened on Saturday . . .
other than I worked out and at night I was chilling in the dorm
with a bunch of people and I coughed up a lot of blood (like
maybe 45 ccs), and then coughed up more blood at like 3:00
a.m., so I had to stop treatments, and I've been getting worse
since then. And now my lungs feel horrible . . . congested, deep
mucus that I can't get out, irritated lungs from trying. I've got
shortness of breath, blood-tinged mucus, etc. I couldn't sleep
last night because I was up coughing.

My lack of sleep has made me tense and irritable and overly
sensitive to things, and Dr. Weill says that if the oral antibiotic
Levaquin doesn't work, then he might want to do IVs, which
would be TERRIBLE. It would be the ultimate failure. I don't
get it. I do everything right, everything, and I even gain weight

(I'm over 150 again—ew), and I still get worse and worse. It's not even that I can't get my pulmonary function test (PFT) up to 3.4 liters—if I got back to that I would be saying hallelujah and thanking God. But I just keep declining despite the fact that I'm doing everything right.

I'm learning that you can't just go through the motions with treatment and all the medicines and everything. It has to BE YOUR LIFE. It can't be just part of life. Inevitably, if you don't make it your life, then you just get sick again. Whenever I'm having the most fun in my life, my health is the worst, which obviously makes everything stop being fun. Because when you don't feel well, nothing else can make you happy.

I got pulled over by the police and got a bike ticket today for running through a stop sign and I just started bawling because I was so overwhelmed and so hot and so tired and feeling so sick and just so behind in everything, and they probably thought I was a crazy stupid little girl who thinks a bike ticket is a huge issue but it wasn't about that. I had been on my way to class but I just turned around and went straight back to the dorm and cried for a while and coughed up a bunch of mucus and almost threw up and then I got on the floor on the carpet with my face right up to the fan in order to cool down for like ten minutes, and then I realized how pathetic I was being and I got myself up and changed clothes and went to class and was late.

10/9/11

It's been a month since I've been back at school. What a whirl-wind!

I switched majors from Earth Systems to HumBio!* It was such a crazy decision, but a good one. I was starting to have all

* Human Biology at Stanford

these doubts about Earth Systems and the hard sciences and math required. HumBio is awesome because it's Evolution, Ecology, Environmental Sciences, Anthropology, Biology, History, etc. It's a ton of stuff all wrapped up together. Other than the core, I'm also taking an Anthropology class called Social and Environmental Sustainability. It's going to be a ton of work but I like it. And every reading so far has made me feel like a smarter person and more educated in fields I actually care about.

I've been doing masters swimming and I LOVE it. The coach is super nice . . . I go every Monday, Wednesday, and Friday. I'm really happy that I planned that into my schedule and have been able to stick with it. I've actually gotten in pretty great shape compared to last year. I go to the gym a lot, too, and one day I even ran six miles. I was definitely sweating but I wasn't dying or anything.

I've been going to club volleyball Tuesday and Thursday nights. Our team is going to be a lot more cohesive this year, and it's nice to be involved in the decisions of the team and in setting the tone of the team.

11/19/11

Had a couple of crazy breakdowns and panic attacks. I've been on an emotional roller coaster for weeks. It's my fifteenth day in Stanford Hospital. I've been here since Nov. 4. As it usually happens, I got admitted for a decline in lung function.

One night I stayed in and cried and drew a picture of me and Micah and felt lonely cuz I missed him. That night I broke down and called my parents and they said to quit something, so I quit my job as an assistant coach. The night of Nov. 3 I broke down but didn't call them and instead was just sobbing in the lounge thinking nobody would understand. Then emailed for a pulmonary function test (PFT) and got admitted the next day.

People who have visited—it shows me who my true friends are. Who doesn't come at all or do anything or even know? Who comes once and that's enough? Who comes all the time and keeps in touch and makes me feel like they miss me? Life is going on without me. . . .

11/22/11

I feel like I'm a fly caught in a spider's web, and the more I struggle to get free, the more tightly I'm trapped and the more quickly I accelerate my demise. The web is CF, but it's also my own emotions about growing up, changing, facing the disease with dignity. It's the difficulty of finding balance between being carefree and being responsible. It's learning how to treat the disease with the respect it deserves without making it the focal point of my life, ruining my personality, or allowing it to drown me.

I don't know why I'm so afraid of EVERYTHING. All of a sudden. I'm afraid of being myself, I think (which makes me worry too much about how people perceive me). I worry that no one will ever love me (which might seem ridiculous, but if I can't love myself, how could someone else?). I worry that I'm losing who I am and losing the ability to have fun. I fear that I'm succumbing to depression (or bipolar disorder? or just insane mood swings which don't really show externally but eat at me from the inside?). I fear that the choices I make are going to cut my life short. Would I rather live a long life and modify my expectations for how that life will look? Or would I rather have the "go hard or go home" mentality and go all out, love life, have fun, live like everyone else, not look back, and accept that what happens, happens?

I just don't think I can do that. Because if I don't feel well, I'll always be sad and afraid and then I'll just spend more and more

time on IVs and in the hospital. Fear that if I can't drink anymore—
because apparently now I'm going to be on voriconazole (an anti-
fungal) for the rest of my life, and it's very hard on the liver, so
drinking is a big risk—then I won't enjoy college because everyone drinks, I won't be happy, I won't have friends or a relationship, and I'll just be that sick girl.

Self-doubt because it feels like I literally can't handle ANY-
THING that's put on me anymore, everything stresses me out.
Even PACKING for Thanksgiving stresses me out. I feel like all
the threads of my life are just unraveling and I'm standing here
helplessly watching it happen and can't do anything about it. And
I'm paralyzed inside my own head and don't know what the right
decisions are.

My mom always says indecisiveness is a sign of insecurity,
because you don't trust yourself to make the right decisions. I
think that's what is happening to me. I don't trust myself to prioritize my time correctly. What's more important? Eating? Sleeping? Treatment? Exercise? Social time? When I give in to the
temptation of living a normal life, I sacrifice time I should be
spending doing treatment because I want to be with people,
whether that means eating or working out or doing homework or
partying/drinking or hanging out. It's so hard to choose sleep or
treatment when that means closing the door on developing relationships that I want to pursue because I want to feel connected
to this school and to other people.

I don't understand why I feel so lonely . . . I have had so
many friends come to visit me here, they show me that they care
so much, they seem to love me, and yet I just don't feel like
anyone knows me. They care, but it doesn't torment them that
I'm here . . . but why should it? Their lives just go on . . . while
mine stops. I'm stuck here, and I'm not getting better, and everything stagnates. And everything in the outside world just keeps

happening. Developing friendships was such a huge goal of mine for this year, branching out, making new friends that aren't just acquaintances.

When I'm stuck in the hospital I can't meet anyone new, I can't participate in campus life, I feel like I'm going to fade away and be forgotten. And then when I'm back I'll just be some random girl who no one knows and who doesn't really know very many people. I want to feel connected to the community of Stanford.

12/19/11

I'm home for Christmas break. Got here on Friday, today is Monday. I don't think I've ever been so happy to be home, to just hang out, be around my parents and Maria and Micah, to have the time and space to stretch out and be alone but also to be with people I care about. Not to be under pressure all the time and not to feel the *need* to do anything.

This last quarter has been hard. I'm going to be on IVs for three to six months, which is a bit funny (well not really funny, more like ironic? A sad twist? Fated? Something I should have seen coming?) considering they told me when I got admitted that first time on November 4 that I would either be doing seven, fourteen, or twenty-one days of IVs max.

I did those first three weeks, sucked it up, first two were in the hospital, then I went home for Thanksgiving, but I had terrible reactions to drugs and felt like absolute shit. Headaches, nausea *all the time,* to the point that it was completely debilitating, I was exhausted, I had no energy, no appetite. I was not myself at all. Wednesday of Thanksgiving break, I had heart palpitations, so I went to Dr. Roston (Dr. Pornchai left Cedars, so I am using my parents' doctor) and he did some tests, but after conferring with Stanford, they decided I was okay and so we pulled the PICC line out. I was nervous to go back to school but also hoping things had turned around.

I went back to Stanford on Sunday, then playing volleyball that Tuesday night was almost physically painful because I was coughing so much and it was that frustrating cough that's so unproductive where you can't get anything up but you just can't stop, and you just can't get enough air, so nothing moves.

Wednesday I woke up with a terrible chest pain, every time I coughed, it hurt, when I breathed in deeply, exhaled deeply. When I did treatment it hurt, when I exerted myself in swimming, it hurt. So I went to the hospital and endured the four-hour clinic wait (terrible when there's no Wi-Fi or phone service and I was way too exhausted and apathetic and upset and pissed and sick of everything to do work).

When I was finally in the room with Dr. Mohabir he said I needed to get admitted. I wasn't happy about this but I trust him. A co-director of the Center for Advanced Lung Disease at Stanford, he's THE *B. cepacia* expert on the West Coast who happens to be a Canadian workout junkie and ex-archaeologist. On his days *off*, he's in the hospital from 6:00 a.m. to 5:00 p.m.; this man puts the Energizer Bunny to shame. I trust him and I love him.

He wanted me for "observation." Twenty-four hours max, he said at first but then changed it to forty-eight hours. But no IVs. Just to have a heart monitor, make sure the chest pain wasn't life threatening. He thought maybe I was having a bad reaction to ataluren, so he took me off it again. I was suspicious but followed orders. There were no beds so I went back to my dorm to get some things. Came back to the intermediate ICU around 9:00-ish. I told my parents not to come since I'd only be there forty-eight hours. Wednesday night and Thursday I watched TV and felt really alone.

My chest X-ray showed that I had developed a cavitation* in
the upper right lobe, which is unusual. They didn't know if it was
a pneumonia (bacterial) or a fungal infection; the X-ray doesn't
give all the details. So we did a CT scan,** which was also somewhat inconclusive. They decided to do a bronchoscopy, so my
mom flew up. But then the day of, they canceled because they
realized that with what happened after the last bronch it's too risky.
Instead they chose to treat the cavitation as a fungal infection and
impressed upon me how serious it was. It was causing pleuritic
chest pain, which means that the fungus was growing up against
the lung wall. It's the kind of thing where if you don't treat it early
enough, it can grow out of control and never go away. And a certain type of fungus is particularly fast growing, and renders you
ineligible for lung transplant (immunosuppressants required post-
transplant would allow the fungus to spread and kill you quickly).

I realized this was serious, and they said I had to get another
PICC line to do four weeks minimum of IV antifungals. They
wanted to treat the ABPA*** with the prednisone and continue the
voriconazole, because my IgE**** was still rising (a normal person's
is like 200, mine in November at first was 1,004, and then it went
up to 1,300), which showed that I wasn't responding to the treatments, so they had to be more aggressive. The IV antifungals
would also fight the cavitation.

I didn't feel better after I started these treatments. They sent
me home after four days, meds in tow, and I resumed my life
(kind of). I worked out moderately, had home health nurses, went
to class when I felt up to it, hung out with friends, etc. But I
wasn't feeling better and the nausea continued.

* A thick-walled gas-filled space within the lung
** a computerized tomography scan that provides more information than an X-ray
*** allergic bronchopulmonary aspergillosis
**** antibodies produced by the immune system

Got through finals with major difficulty. Extremely exhausted, worried, feeling like a failure. But I did my presentation, finished my entire paper, took two HumBio finals. Then went to clinic for the follow-up and found out that my IgE had risen to 1,800. Ugh, still climbing. Also, white blood count was too high, about 16,000, which shows a bacterial infection going on, too. My chest X-ray showed that the infiltration/cavitation was growing, not going away, which I knew because I could still feel tightness.

They told me that doctors from Stanford (adult and pediatric), from Denmark, from Toronto, etc., had collaborated about my case, that they had presented it to the national conference or something because it was so complex, and they decided that they needed to treat all three problems at once—the ABPA, the fungal infection, and the B. cepacia infection—each aggressively. They decided on three to six months of IV antibiotics and antifungals, oral antibiotics and antifungals, and prednisone. They asked me if I was willing to do this, and I said of course I was, but of course I started crying as I realized what that really meant.

Giving up club volleyball and masters swimming is upsetting, but also giving up on sleep with middle-of-the-night IVs. It's giving up on showers, on feeling carefree, on having the luxury to worry about things like classes. It's knowing that I'm not going to feel comfortable getting close to a guy because I have way too much baggage—no one will want that. And sex with a PICC line and an IV drip?

It's knowing that I won't be able to relate to my friends because their gossip and their concerns will be so mundane to me. It's realizing that I can't put my toes in the sand, go for a long run and sweat out all my toxins, can't take a super long shower and let the water run over me. Losing simple things that everyone takes for granted represents more loss.

They also pulled me from the ataluren trial permanently. I left the final appointment with Colleen and Zoe★ quickly because I was embarrassed to be crying as we said our goodbyes. I get really embarrassed about all these emotions, especially with my mom because she always says I never let any of this stuff get me down, like that's what makes me a role model and inspirational to people. And I do want to try to keep my head up through these things, I think I have been able to do that, despite the adversity. BUT you can't just ignore things, sweep them under the rug. People keep telling me that I'll adjust. They just don't understand what it's like to have your life ripped away from you because they don't realize the things I have to give up when I'm on IVs. And when it's just for a short time, it's like I'm just taking a vacation from those things—from being in the water, from playing volleyball, from bike riding, from everything, really. And not only can I not do all of these things that keep me sane, I have all of these worries that are exacerbated when I'm on IVs. I'm hyperaware of my breathing, of how much I'm coughing, how much mucus I have, which I can never move because I can't exercise. I'm always tired, I get wiped out, my stomach has issues because of all the hardcore drugs, I have to have a freaking PICC line in my arm, which is pretty isolating because it's strange and intimidating to people. And now I have three IV drugs that I'm taking on top of the oral voriconazole and an oral antibiotic which I haven't picked up from the pharmacy yet . . . gahhh, and prednisone, plus all the stuff I was already taking before (including my long treatments).

I'm going to stop wallowing. I'm home for break . . . want to enjoy it while it lasts, and try not to think about how difficult the

---

★ Colleen Dunn and Zoe Davies were the research manager and research coordinator, respectively, of the clinical trial. Mallory adored them.

next quarter or two will be. I just need to take it one day at a time. Stretch a lot. Shower around the PICC and keep myself well-groomed so I feel good about myself. Try to just be myself and be outgoing and seem happy to other people and maybe I'll convince myself that I'm not so sad and forget that I might even be scared. I'm living a double life right now, the life that goes on when I'm with my parents and with the doctors and doing treatment (the life of someone with a SERIOUS illness and serious complications), and the life of Mallory Smith, a student, a friend, an athlete, maybe to someone a girl of potential interest, or maybe just that tall girl out there who seems just like everyone else, who goes to class, goes out to eat, goes to parties, goes to the gym, does homework, etc. It's so funny the things about you that people miss when they just pay attention to your actions and not your thoughts, how much that way of assessing someone conceals.

It's so nice to be home. I've been sleeping a lot and adjusting to this crazy IV schedule. And hanging out with high school friends, who I've missed SO MUCH. Dewey* has arthritis and seems in pain. Why is so much falling apart, my body, my dog's body, my sense of meaning in the crazy scheme of this entire planet?

2012

1/2/12
It's just so freaking HARD figuring out how to live, because the docs always say not to let CF hold you back, do everything you

---

* the family dog

want to do, and figure out how to work treatments and health stuff in, but it doesn't work that way. With CF if you want to be healthy and live a long time, you have to devote your entire body and soul to it; you can't devote yourself to normal things that your peers do and find time for health. Squeezing everything in just doesn't work. Planning to go abroad is futile, I'm just setting myself up for disappointment, or maybe I could get there but I'd make myself sicker in the long run and accelerate my decline.

I can't plan things that other people plan. Like weekend getaways. I can't plan to party and still do well in school. To travel to third-world countries and do something of significance. To go camping. To get married and have kids. I can't imagine letting anyone understand the way my body actually works, because I find it disgusting and revolting, so I wouldn't want anyone except my parents and doctors to understand.

3/15/12

I'm so pissed at OAE. They just don't get how hard my life is. Instead of writing what happened, I'm going to paste in my email exchange with them, so I remember.

> To:<—@stanford.edu>
> Sent: Monday, March 12, 2012 9:41:40 PM
>
> I was wondering if I could set up a meeting to discuss my grading for Spanish this quarter. I understand the problem in that I have not followed the attendance policy, but I do feel that I can make up work that would allow me to practice/learn whatever was done in class on the days that I have missed—doing a final presentation this week, completing the take-home

quiz, watching the movie and writing a summary/
mini-essay about it, doing practice exercises on the
book's website that correspond to the days I missed,
and if this is not enough, recording myself having
conversation with a native Spanish speaker for however
long would be required to make up the conversation
time I missed in class.

Thank you so much,

* * *

From:<—@stanford.edu>
Sent: Tuesday, March 13, 2012 7:32:00 PM
Subject: Re: meeting

Hi Mallory,
I could meet with you on Friday, but my job as a
coordinator is not to bend the rules but rather to stick
to them. All I'll be able to tell you is that you may take
an incomplete and make up the missed classes next
quarter in Span Lang 15 and/or makeup classes. You
do indeed need to complete the assignments you cite
below, but in addition you need a total of 27–30 hours
of attendance to pass the class. That is the basic rule for
the class, even under difficult circumstances.

I'm so sorry, Mallory, that I can't offer you an
easier option, but I'm happy to support you in any way
possible to make the "makeup" process doable for you.

Best,

* * *

To:<—@stanford.edu>
Sent: Wednesday, March 14, 2012 2:34 AM

I don't mean to offend you, and maybe I am just not
understanding why there is absolutely NO way for me
to finish the class this quarter, but I find it borderline
discriminatory that I may be prevented from taking
language classes ever again at Stanford because of this
attendance policy. At the beginning of each quarter,
when I sign up for classes, I cannot predict what
health hurdles will come my way—I don't know how
often I will be spending nights in the ER, how many
days I will be in the hospital, or how many appointments I will need to schedule with doctors who have
hundreds of patients and can't accommodate my class
schedule in their scheduling. Since it seems that there
is no way for you to bend the rules in this extenuating
circumstance, the implication is that I cannot take
language classes at this school. At this point, I believe
it would be very detrimental to my health next
quarter to have lingering responsibilities from this
quarter. I am inclined to say that maybe I should just
take the fail in the class if my only options are a fail or
an incomplete. I've never faced an attendance policy
that was absolutely unable to be modified in any
circumstance. I don't think we need to meet on Friday
just for you to tell me that I can only get an incomplete, so I'm just going to think about what to do and
then get back to you.

* * *

From: "Diane Shader Smith"
To: "Mallory Beatrice Smith"
Sent: Wednesday, March 14, 2012 6:00:52 AM

XXX is only a lecturer, not the dean or a higher up. You're protected from this discrimination by the Americans with Disabilities Act. I will find language that you can send to them. In the meantime you should email the CF team for documentation about your hospitalizations. xo

* * *

It all worked! Issue resolved. They agreed not to count my missed days, so I passed the class!

4/30/12

My PICC line is the emblem of the chains holding me back, a burning, unyielding reminder of the losses of my present and the uncertainties of my future. Not a minute of respite or peaceful freedom can be won until I'm released from the tethering leash that holds me hostage within a life restricted, a cage that feels far too small.

5/29/12

I dream that one day CF will stand for Cure Found. I dream that one day breathing will become so easy that I could take it for granted, although I never will.

6/7/12

Want to apply for a CF merit grant. Need to list my accomplishments at Stanford to date:

- Outreach chair—Health Advocacy Program
- Research assistant—Stanford Food Project
- Member—Students for Sustainable Stanford
- Member—Appetite for Change

What I care about: raising awareness about the environment and ethical and health issues associated with meat consumption and the food industry. Specifically, the intersection between human societies and the environment, and sustainable development and agriculture.

6/25/12

Finally figured out that I wanted to plan for a career in sustainable development of developing countries and applied for/was accepted into a program to work in a remote town in Ecuador. But with my unrelenting pneumonia, invasive fungal infection, hemoptysis, ABPA, gallstones, and a pulmonary embolism, my doctors immediately nixed the plan.

I was devastated. While I moped, my mom, in classic form, swooped in and figured out a plan B better than my plan A—a nine-week environmental documentary filmmaking program at UC Santa Barbara called "Blue Horizons." The application was intense but now I'm in S.B.!

Got here yesterday in time for my orientation, then moved into my housing. My housemates are really nice! Need to decorate my room since it's pretty barren. Excited for this program but nervous about the time commitment, the workload, getting enough sleep, treatment and exercise.

6/27/12

Today we had a field trip to Coal Oil Point Reserve, a nature reserve near campus. I walked over with Ashley who is super nice, and we decided to do the documentary project together. We were scheming about who else we wanted to work with and decided on Spencer and Nick. Today we approached Nick on the hike through the reserve. He said he was down to be in our group, so

now we just have to ask Spencer. It's amazing how much information the program has covered in three days. Finally got into the
ocean! First time since I came to Santa Barbara . . .

6/30/12

The long hours and group work make me feel close to the people in the program even though I've only known them for six
days. It's amazing to me that one week ago I didn't know one
person in Santa Barbara and now I feel connected to Ashley,
Nick, and Spencer!

We had a camera-handling workshop from 10:00 to 2:00.
INTERESTING!

7/2/12

GOOD THINGS THAT HAPPENED TODAY:

1. Turned in my rental camera equipment—had been worried
about forgetting or oversleeping
2. Took a nap, went to yoga at S.B. yoga center again, made it to
CVS for meds
3. Came up with cool idea for video pitch to send to pharmaceutical companies about handling life as a young adult with
CF—things the docs don't tell you—and use Blue Horizons
equipment to shoot footage that I can use later
4. Ate really delicious and healthy breakfast: nonfat Greek yogurt with dried cherries, chia seeds, sunflower seeds, organic
wildflower honey, raspberries and blueberries, and blonde roast
Starbucks coffee ☺
5. Matt (a housemate) invited me to play beach volleyball tomorrow afternoon, which should be fun if I can still play after
not playing for so long and feeling out of shape

BAD/MEH THINGS THAT HAPPENED TODAY:

1. Zoned out for a half hour of our three-hour Final Cut Pro workshop
2. Had really bad period cramps and stomach issues today, drank Cathy's PMS relief herbs. They have mugwort in them haha
3. Didn't sleep enough last night so really exhausted all day

7/26/12

Went to clinic today. My IgE went from 700 to 569 (so much better than the high of 2,400 last December), my liver enzymes are continuing to drop toward normal range, my blood sugar is good, so no diabetes. The bad news is that my heart rate continues to be higher than normal and I'm more short of breath/ my energy is still lower than it should be. White count is also elevated, which confirms my suspicions that what's going on is increased infection, leading to more mucus clogging, difficulty breathing, low energy, high heart rate, etc. I'm just fucking pissed about it because I only got off of IVs six weeks ago, and I started feeling this new infection, whatever is going on now, about two weeks ago; that means I had four weeks of freedom, and that doesn't seem fair. I don't know what I'm doing wrong, and I don't want to talk to my mom about it because she will say that I need to slow down, to do less, etc., but I can't right now. I'm not a perfectionist or an overachiever but I just can't right now.

When I'm healthy, IT'S A BEAUTIFUL THING, and I feel like I'm capable of anything: I'm motivated, happy, spontaneous, energetic, and fun. When I'm sick, I'm none of those things. If I lived my life like a sick person, always limiting what I think I'm capable of and limiting what I do so that I never get sick, then I would have all the negative consequences of being sick in addition to the physical feeling of it. I just don't know what to do and it's stressing me out and making me sad and I can foresee my future self absolutely hating me, screaming, "Why the fuck did you care about this whale movie so much? The rest of the group could have picked up your slack!!" But I can't explain why I can't NOT do what I came here to do. It's REALLY stressful making a film and taking it way too seriously.

8/22/12

Silver Bullet turned out to be a great film but so much drama in our group when we were finishing. I am proud of it but the shit storm at the end probably compromised my health. It sucks but I really loved the program and learned so much. Sad to have it end.

8/29/12

I was chosen to be a Peer Health Educator (PHE) in Cedro dorm, a job I really wanted but wasn't sure I'd be healthy enough to do! We're responsible for the health and wellness of the freshmen in our dorm, but people joke that the real job is to pass out condoms.

9/16/12

Turns out the stress of balancing the PHE job with my health needs feels like an infection in its own right, wreaking havoc on my physical and emotional health. In the first few days certain coworkers did not understand the severity of my condition and seemed to feel that I was trying to shirk my work responsibilities. They had no idea what my life is like. But our dynamic became instantly better after I sent a long, heartfelt email explaining.

9/18/12

I'm back in the hospital thinking about what I want:

I want to wake up in the morning and take a deep, full breath.

I want that breath to fill me up, to imbue me with joy and energy, not to irritate or pain me and set off a spasm of coughing.

I want to be able to do the things that I dream of while I sleep, things that are taxing in reality: hiking, running, biking, swimming, diving, kicking, screaming, dancing, laughing, jumping, falling, leaping, soaring. . . .

I want to get to know another person without fearing what they will think when they *truly* understand the way my body works.

I want to trust that my body will be able to help me, not hinder me, in living out my dreams.

I want to know that when my closest friends are sitting on the porch at age eighty, I'll be sitting there with them, reminiscing, smiling, weeping, talking, drifting, chuckling.

I want to fall in love and have a relationship that's reciprocal, and not have to burden my love with the task of taking care of a spouse who can't pull her own weight, who's *needy*.

I want to have a child, but more than that, I want to *hope* to have a child without the nagging worry that the dream is entirely foolish. And when I have this child, I want to be able to pick her up, carry her around, chase after her in the playground, climb trees with her, play with her in the jungle gym, teach her how to swim, dance with her in the kitchen, show her the most beautiful hikes, be there to push her into her first wave, keep up with her fireball energy of youth.

I want to effect change in the world. I want my life goals not to end at solely surviving.

I want to live largely, richly, vastly, dynamically, lovingly, graciously, eternally, and ephemerally.

I want to feel amazement and wonder, every day.

I want to never lose sight of my place in the thread of humanity, in the fabric of the earth, in the palace that is this universe.

I want friendship, happiness, humor, laughter, lightheartedness, small conquerable worries.

To want these things is normal; to expect them is dangerous.

Do I have to abandon my beautiful idea of what life is? Do I have to abandon these fantasies as possibilities for me, to refashion my idea of the future, to settle for just surviving, breath by breath, one day at a time, sacrificing the very idea of dreams to prevent disappointment?

Only if I allow disappointment to crush my spirit.

I am happy today.

10/19/12

Things have been going better for me. I'm on top of my shit and having fun. But I did have a moment of realization that I don't want to do my major anymore. Maybe it was a temporary freak-out but I used to envision doing environmental work in the field outside all day and working with people, doing photography or filmmaking or research or education or outreach or whatever. Now I just see those careers being too physically hard and since I can't know what I'll be capable of in the future, it seems silly to plan for a career that might not work for me. What led me to study the environment in the first place might never be feasible and I don't want to end up doing physically easy things like administration, office work, etc.

2013

2/17/13

The tournament at Davis was so fun! I got to see Michelle and play lots of volleyball. And drive home with Karen with the music blasting! Saturday night my mom treated our team to dinner at the Spaghetti Factory, and even though I ate to the point of feeling physically ill half the night, it was great.

Everyone was grateful that my mom paid for dinner, but it makes me feel ashamed about the fact that I couldn't go to these tournaments and do okay without her. I guess ashamed isn't the right word. Embarrassed? No. It's not really about admitting to other people that I need her, it's about admitting it to myself. I don't really know what I'm saying. I'm happy she comes, it allows me to play, but I wish I had the luxury of being like the other girls on the team whose parents can just show up during the daytime to watch them play every so often, instead of needing a parent to fly up north, drive up with me in advance, stay in the room with me, pack for me, clean my gear for me, get me breakfast, watch me all day and get me food and drinks, pay for dinner so she can justify coming with the team. I hate feeling so dependent, but I am.

3/20/13

It's funny how over the years my wishes have evolved, like what I say in my head when my eyes are closed and I'm blowing out the candles, or when I'm in the passenger seat of a car driving through a tunnel, or when I see a shooting star. When I was young I wished for specific things: for someone to have a crush on me, to get to go on a trip, to receive something material that I wanted, to win the respect of a coach and earn a starting spot, etc. Then I would just wish to be healthy, nice and simple. Then it was, "I wish to be healthy and *happy*." The second half was added on because that was starting to feel unobtainable. Now, it's just, "I wish to be happy." The most achievable of all, something I used to wake up feeling and take for granted. Now I know that at the most basic level, I need to be happy or I'll never be healthy, mentally or physically.

5/12/13

Today was a really lovely day!

Yesterday, after I got my PICC line out, I wanted to go swimming but wasn't allowed to get my arm wet yet, so I walked the "Dish" at Stanford with Pidge and Uncle Danny. Was nice to spend time with them but I couldn't do the full hike; the heat was killing me more than the workout itself, and I felt very faint and unwell. So, I left them to find someplace to sit and ended up at Tresidder* because I wanted shade and comfort.

Then last night was the Relay for Life. We got there during the opening ceremony and watched the video slideshow in honor of cancer patients. It was SO sad. During the third performance I was bawling as I listened to a sophomore talk about her best friend at Stanford who got diagnosed with brain cancer spring quarter freshman year and died winter quarter of sophomore year. I just couldn't imagine the absolute devastation and despair that everyone who knew her must have felt, what her family must have felt, how she felt when she got the diagnosis. I was imagining these things and it made me feel so hollow, but also so appreciative of my situation, that I have time. But it also made me think about what it would be like if I died, how someone could be standing on a stage at some point, with a candle, talking about what it was like to lose me.

* one of two main hubs where students hang out

And I thought about what my family would be without me, how there would just be this void, and how they've all worked so hard and given up so much for me, how I'm an attention-sucking person because my parents have to sacrifice so much time to make sure that I'm okay, and how they do it in a heartbeat, instinctively, without any second-guessing or hesitation. And if I died, all that effort would just be . . . there's no word for it. They've poured heart and soul, every single bit of emotion they have into keeping me alive, and if I died, all that would die with me. I think my family would feel dead, not forever, they might come back, but it makes me heartsick to think about what I would leave behind if I passed on.

After the ceremony was over there was a silent walk around the track. The whole experience was very emotional. I felt this wave of gratitude at the beauty and magnitude of the human experience, that I get to live; and I felt frustration with myself for so often getting bogged down in the silliest things.

Today I went for a swim at Oak Creek—it was sunny and beautiful, the pool was the perfect temperature, there were a bunch of adorable babies and children, I was able to get some exercise, and SWIM for the first time in weeks! It's always the best way to celebrate getting the PICC line out . . . and it always feels like the very essence of freedom.

11/13/13
I am in Hawaii! Long story short, I was sick last week. First Sabrina got sick, then I started feeling feverish and fatigued, then my stomach got fucked up, and by Wednesday I felt like I was in the middle of a full-blown exacerbation. Crazy how it happens so quickly.

My mom arrived on Tuesday. It ended up being really good timing that she was there while I was sick. I scheduled an appt to go to clinic on Friday, my PFTs were at 42 percent again, down from 52 percent. That's a pretty significant drop, but I wasn't really surprised, because I was so short of breath I could barely even bike to class.

Their strategy for people in my category of health seems to be that when we say we're not feeling well and schedule a clinic appt outside of a regular checkup, we should be admitted, because it's based 99 percent on our stated symptoms and how we feel, not on PFTs or white blood count or anything. Whereas when I was healthier, and I didn't feel that big of a difference between a lung function of 75 percent and 65 percent, they would have to force me to be admitted and I would never choose it voluntarily. But I really did not want to be admitted, I was kind of hoping they would suggest to just watch it, maybe start an oral or something.

Since my right lung sounded junky and my lung function had dropped, they were pushing for admission. My mom popped out with, "Can she go to Hawaii instead?" It caught me off guard but what was more surprising was they said yes. And all of a sudden it was settled!

It feels like I picked myself up out of one life and planted myself in another. I was in the middle of the quarter (week 8) frustrated by the amount of work and meetings and projects and nervous about a midterm, and now all of that has just fallen by the wayside. I brought some work with me but I feel way less stressed and think R and R accelerates the healing process.

The trip has been incredible so far. I'm here with my dad (my mom was busy with work) and it's been wonderful. We're staying at the Royal Hawaiian in Waikiki, which is a change from Wailea. Hoping to meet young people since I didn't bring a friend. Every day I get up and do treatment, then we have breakfast (usually at the café across the street, honey latte and açai bowl), then go down to the beach, and I surf for an hour or so, then relax by the pool, then back in the ocean, come up for a second treatment, and after that either go back down for more ocean/pool time or I go into town for yoga or Pilates. It's been restful and healing, and great quality time with Pidge.

There's a very cute surfboard rental guy who started chatting with me yesterday when I was taking a board out . . . he gave me some of his wax and offered advice about which boards were good. He seems shy but so sweet.

Today my dad and I had tea and coffee at the restaurant by the pool since I wasn't feeling well enough to surf in the morning (nausea), and I was looking for him and kept seeing him wandering around and I saw him go out with a board but couldn't figure out how to go up to him. Around 2:30 I rented a board and was paddling out and saw him paddling in from afar (it looked like he was giving some girl a lesson). He waved at me!

Later, when I was done surfing, I went over to the towel place where he was stationed to chat more. He was looking at footage of dolphins he took on a GoPro while surfing, so we talked about that for a bit, but then he had to get back to work. I'm going to try to go out earlier tomorrow morning, and surf before treatment at 9:00, and maybe he'll be out there and I can talk to him! It's nice to have someone cute in the same age range to talk to, even if it's nothing more than that.

11/17/13

This trip has had a couple of surprising turns of events.

Made progress with Shawn! I finally learned his name. Every day I would see him at the stand where he works, or in the water, but usually just say a few words and smile, because he was busy with work. I would also see him while he was giving lessons and we would wave at each other. Finally, yesterday he came up to me in the water on his board (he was the photographer that day, not the surf instructor, so he had more time to chill once he finished with the photos) and we had a pretty long conversation. It turned out to be an incredible week—we actually went night surfing!

SO bummed to go home. Going back to schoolwork, obligations, no ocean, no boys I'm interested in . . . I mean, I'll be happy once I'm there. But this was the most incredible way of decompressing, getting healthy once again, expanding my comfort zone (by hanging out myself so much and putting myself out there to meet people—I also made other friends on the beach), improving my surfing, proving to myself and others that the ocean really does heal me.

12/8/13

I'm finally processing a traumatic event that happened at the end of September, and am ready to write about it:

I lay on a stretcher in an ambulance, watching as familiar places on campus blurred past the window: the eucalyptus forests I used to be able to run through, the looming trees lining Palm Drive, my freshman dorm, the gym where I played volleyball. The paramedic scribbled notes and my hands clutched a huge stack of paper towels that were saturated with the caked blood that had been inside me just a few minutes before. With quick, shallow breaths, I tried to take in air without bursting any more fragile blood vessels in my scarred airways.

Arriving at the ER, I was whisked past the long line of waiting patients into a private room. The nature of my emergency demanded that I be ushered straight in, bypassing the waiting room and the triage station.

My parents met me in the room. They stroked my hair, looking worried.

"Thank God we didn't go home yet," my mom said. "What if we had already left?"

As if my mom would leave when I was still sick . . .

The pulmonologist on call came into my room. "So," he began, in a somber tone, "why don't you tell me what happened?"

"I moved back to school two weeks ago, and three days later was admitted to the hospital for a severe lung function decline," I explained. "I've been on triple IV antibiotic therapy since then. I was released two days ago to move back to the dorm and continue IV therapy there. Tonight I woke up at 2:00 a.m., needing to cough. I could feel the blood pooling in my lungs. I coughed up about a half a cup of blood. It felt like it was never going to stop."

I didn't say that when I woke up, my first coherent thought had been that an episode of hemoptysis was coming. I didn't tell the doctor how I'd grabbed the paper towels by my bedside as blood surged up into my throat, or how, not wanting to stain the bed, I'd rolled onto the floor and stayed there, coughing up blood. How each inhalation had brought more of the sticky red; no breath, no matter how shallow, felt safe. Moving was impossible; it would have deepened my breaths and worsened the situation, so I'd remained on my side, aware, between coughs, of the cold-ness and hardness of the wood floor. I felt like I was drowning. Knowing I'd have to report the quantity of blood to the doctors, I spread paper towels across the floor to absorb it. The white squares were splattered with pools of blood, resembling a morbid piece of modern art.

When I could feel the flood subside a bit, I staggered to my desk to call 9-1-1. Breathless, I explained the emergency and re-quested that an ambulance be dispatched immediately. The woman on the phone did not understand that every question she asked me to answer caused more rupturing and more blood. Our one-minute conversation felt painfully long and drawn out. When she finally agreed to send an ambulance, I hung up, then texted my parents to meet me at the ER.

The doctor took notes as I talked and asked the usual questions about my medical history. There was nothing he could do but admit me and so I was wheeled on my gurney to a real room. It was crushing to be back in so soon; I had hoped I might get at least a couple of months of respite.

A few hours later, Dr. Mohabir came to see me.

"This is really serious, Mallory," he said, standing at the foot of my bed in his yellow isolation gown. "Sub-massive bleeds almost always result in massive bleeds soon after. We'll keep you another week for observation. No food or water for forty-eight hours, in case we need to do surgery. No treatments; your airways need to rest. Take it very easy." And then, because he knew that the school year was about to start, "I know this is bad timing, but this is a life-threatening emergency."

12/9/13

It's interesting that after all these years there's one word everyone uses to describe daily therapy—treatment. My dad used to call it Pat Pat as part of the game he called Astronaut and Pat Pat to help me be okay with the manual therapy they started on me at the age of three. I hated when he'd pound my chest to loosen the mucus so I used to hide. I came to understand that my dad created a game and my mom wrote *Mallory's 65 Roses* to help me understand why I had to do treatment every day.*

When I was five I got my first vest to do chest percussion therapy (CPT). Now, as an outpatient, I do it two to three times

* I wrote *Mallory's 65 Roses,* a children's picture book illustrated by Disney animator Jay Jackson, to explain what the disease was and all that it entailed. We read it to her class at the start of each school year, gave a copy to each of her friends, and had it distributed nationwide since there was then no educational material about CF for young children. Mallory became somewhat of a celebrity, her friends and their families accepted the diagnosis, and life was okay.

a day for about two hours in total. Inpatient protocol calls for CPT four times a day. My vest is a black (it also comes in pink) inflatable ensemble that shakes the bloody hell out of my lungs, mobilizes mucus, and looks ridiculous. During this loud and strange-looking ritual, I also inhale four medications back to back through a nebulizer, which many bewildered and envious college students have mistaken for a vaporizer. My outpatient machines give me a look that combines astronaut-launching-into-space with fierce-policewoman-wearing-bulletproof-vest.

As an inpatient, a respiratory therapist comes every four hours and does different forms of CPT: sometimes vest; sometimes G5, a black handheld toy that looks like a giant vibrator; sometimes IPV, an aggressive nebulizer that shakes the lungs from inside out; and sometimes manual percussion, which involves the therapist flipping me upside down and beating my chest and back like a drummer at a rock concert for two arduous minutes in each of eight different positions. My method of choice in the hospital is manual percussion because it's not only effective but also hilarious.

These days I still find myself struggling to integrate the implications of this disease and the accompanying complicated medical regimen into my fragmented life, to unify disparate elements from the "real world" and the "sick world" into one cohesive existence. But the world of chronic illness—with mucus, blood, infection, hospitals, and fear—doesn't fit very neatly into the typical college experience—the other world of dorms, meal plans, parties, GPAs, and recklessness.

My life on campus is a parallel universe that I sometimes feel part of, but often not, because of the ticking time bomb inside my body—a bomb that often blows to bits any sense of normalcy. The true home base of my daily reality is Stanford Hospital.

Many people have some notion of a "second home"— a sleepaway camp, their grandparents' house. My second home is

now Stanford Hospital. During my most recent stay, the one that
began with that ambulance ride across campus, I started thinking
about how hospitals, to me, are so much more than a physical
infrastructure; they act as a sort of ad hoc community center for
those of us living in the parallel existence of chronic illness.
Chronic illness interferes with social connections, but it can also
create other, more powerful opportunities for community. In de-
fining my college experience and even my identity, few places
have mattered more than Stanford Hospital.

That morning, when the blinds of my hospital room were
finally opened, I squinted, bleary-eyed, into the unfamiliar eyes of
an unknown man in scrubs. There's some kind of color-coding
system in place to help patients identify the role of each hospital
worker based on the color of their scrubs, but I've yet to figure it
out. This youngish, wiry-framed man identified himself as an interventional radiologist, and while I wrestled with my sheets and
the controls on the bed, trying to sit myself up, he launched into
a speech full of detailed information about the cauterization procedure I would have to undergo if I coughed up any more blood.
My mom gripped the edge of the bed and I saw fear in her eyes.
Groggy and cranky, I couldn't pay attention. Instead, I repeated
orders in my head for him to leave me alone and let me sleep.
Unfortunately, he did not seem to receive my telepathic commands.

When he left, I looked at the clock. Ten o'clock. My first
class of junior year, an economics course, was beginning a short
way away on campus. I imagined the sound of the hourly bells
and pictured myself doing what I should have been doing: waking
up a little earlier than necessary, taking too long to get ready, racing across campus on my bike, walking into class winded and
windblown, grabbing a seat in back. I saw a tear splash on the
sheet before I realized I was crying. Shivering, with my arm hair

standing on end, I buzzed the nurses' station for another blanket.
Hospitals are always so damned cold.

My first two days in-house I was kept busy by doctors and nurses.
I slept, avoided thoughts of food or water, and wondered whether
it was worth the effort to shower. On the third morning I was
finally allowed to eat. This was a big deal because it meant I had
made it past the forty-eight-hour period during which the risk
for a massive hemoptysis episode is highest. To celebrate, I ordered four scrambled eggs with pepper, French toast, yogurt, coffee, pineapple, grapes, and peanut butter. Hospital food had never
tasted so good.

I was also allowed to start CPT again, but gently. I was just as
relieved about this. I hated being caught in the catch-22 of hemoptysis. Hemoptysis is caused by infection, but when it happens, you have to stop doing CPT treatments, which you do to
fight infection. The infection and mucus pooling then worsen,
causing more scarring and rupturing of the airways, eventually
leading to more hemoptysis.

Despite the awkwardness of these bizarre CPT rituals (or perhaps because of it), I've gotten close to many of the respiratory
therapists. That morning Jainko was assigned to my room.
Through her many visits we chat about our favorite teas, books,
and countries while I hyperventilate and try to keep my ribs un-
broken.

Halfway through this first treatment, Martina, one of the
housekeepers, walked in to say hi. *"¡Cómo me alegra verte! ¡Ojalá no
estés muy enferma!"* Translated that means, "Nice to see you, hope
you're not really sick!" During my last visit, Martina had told me
she has three daughters, and one has a derelict boyfriend. She's
cleaned my room every time I've been hospitalized during the

past two years. It's nice to see a familiar face who brings no bad news, just good conversations and compassion.

I awoke early on my fourth day to Dr. Mohabir's signature enthusiastic knock.

"How much longer do I have to stay?" I asked, knowing I probably wouldn't get the answer I wanted. "It's Thursday and I haven't had any hemoptysis since Sunday night."

"We can't rush this. You're still at risk for a major bleed, so I don't want you leaving until I'm confident that it won't happen again right after you leave. That means we have to build up to full force on your CPT, and you have to build up to doing some physical activity while you're here to make sure walking won't trigger another episode."

His words gave me my goal for the day: taking my first walk. My mom yelped with joy; she'd been asking every day since I arrived when she could start forcing me to move. This is a constant battle between us when I'm in the hospital. She has the mindset of the coach of an Olympic athlete and looks to the doctor for backup when I don't want to comply with her walking demands. The doctor tries to stay out of the debate by saying, "Whatever she feels up to doing. She'll know how much is too much." I usually don't fight her anymore—resisting is more draining than the walk itself. But this admission, Dr. Mohabir had said no walking until he gave permission; my mom had been quietly dying inside at my lack of physical activity. The look on her face when she was told she could resume her role as drill sergeant was one of pure joy.

My walk that day didn't go very well. After five minutes I couldn't breathe. Coughing fits are too hard on the lungs when they're fragile, so I had to stop. This was very distressing to my mother. But Dr. Mohabir reassured her, "One day at a time. She's not going from 0 to 180 in a day."

Besides his expertise in B. *cepacia,* one of the reasons I trust Dr. M so much is because he seems to care about me. Once, when I sat in clinic a couple of days after being released from a hospitalization, he could tell I was pretty down. I had just spent a bit of time talking to the social worker about what a hard time I was having, and my eyes were puffy and red-rimmed despite my best efforts to hold back tears. He looked sad for me when I mentioned that I felt physically limited and wasn't optimistic about gaining back my athletic ability.

"What do you want to do, Mal?" he asked. I was puzzled; I didn't really understand the question. "Personally, I just want freedom," he said. "I work out so I can have freedom. A few months ago when I presented my research at the international CF conference in Ireland, I decided afterward to run around Lough Neagh. It's the biggest lake in Ireland, 151 miles around."

I didn't really know where this story was going, but this was the first time he had ever told me something in detail about his personal life. "You just decided to run it? Like straight through without stopping? How long did that take?!" I was absolutely incredulous.

"No, no, not straight through," he responded, chuckling a bit at the thought. "I just put together a light backpack and decided to start running. It took me nine days. I didn't run the entire way. Sometimes I would run for two minutes and get tired and decide to walk for a while. Other times I would run ten miles straight. The point is, I just wanted to be able to see the place in its entirety, and running the perimeter of the lake was the easiest way to do that."

"But . . . where did you sleep?" I had so many logistical questions, I couldn't really focus on the larger point he was trying to make. "Did you pack food and water? A change of clothes?"

"There were places along the way to buy water and food. As

for sleeping, each night I knocked on the door of a friendly-looking house and said, 'I'm a physician from the U.S. here for an international research conference. I'm running around Lough Neagh and I need a place to sleep for the night. I have my own blanket, but can I sleep in your backyard?' Every single person I asked let me come in and insisted that I sleep inside the house instead of the backyard. They all gave me a hearty breakfast in the morning."

I was amazed at the spontaneity of this adventure, but even more amazed by the fact that Dr. Mohabir lives the life I've always dreamed about. My childhood fantasies were peppered with notions of adventure, spontaneity, and simplicity. As I got older and came to understand my dependence on modern technology, electricity, first-world medical facilities, and strict daily schedules, I longed for these fantasies even more. Nothing seemed more appealing to me than living off the grid, without material luxuries, or traveling on a whim, with no dependence on money, people, or places. I'm happy for others when I hear about their adventures, but my genuine happiness is tainted with pangs of jealousy because I'll never be able to do that. CF ties patients to their parents, their treatment schedule, their hospital, and modern technology; freedom, for me, represents the foundation of an unattainable alternate life, the life I would lead if not for CF. After hearing his story, I understood that he was trying to ask: What is it that I want to be able to do with my life? What do I need physical strength *for*?

"I want to be able to travel, to see something other than this bubble that I've grown up in. I want my career to take me into sustainable development of third-world countries. I want to do research in the rain forests of Brazil, to work on an organic coffee farm in Nicaragua, to scuba dive in Australia. I want to be able to hike to the tops of really tall mountains and see what the view's like up there, and to know what it feels like to finish a triathlon, and to be able to spend some time helping the world instead of letting the world help me."

I know he related to those desires, and it was hard for him to deliver what he said next. "Because of your hemoptysis, it's not safe for you to be far from a major medical center for the next few years. But after that, I don't see why you shouldn't be able to do some of these things! Proximity to electricity may be a limiting factor, but I don't think your lung function has to be. I know CF patients out there doing the most amazing things, things they weren't always sure would be possible. Don't give up on those dreams."

Even as he said those words, I knew to take them with a grain of salt. His job is to inspire confidence, and making the impossible seem attainable is a great way to motivate patients to stay happy and continue working hard. His words didn't necessarily convince me that I could live elbow-deep in the soils of Central America for the rest of my life, but they showed that he cared about my future and was going to work with me to make it hold as much promise as possible.

On the fifth morning of that hospitalization, I woke up feeling much better and made up my mind that I would take a significant walk. Outside, the air was crisp and clear, typical of a beautiful Northern California fall day. As my mom and I walked out the door of the front entrance, the sky was clear and the sun hurt my eyes. I squinted and looked down. At the fountain in front of the hospital, ducks paddled around in an incomprehensible social dance. I dipped one foot in the chilly water, wondering whether it ever got cleaned, and then chose to ignore this concern. My second foot followed the first and I sat down on the ledge, ankle-deep in the fountain, goosebumps running up and down my legs.

Craning around to look behind me, I saw my mom point at a girl who was walking a ways away with her dad.

"That girl is in the room next door to you. I've spoken to her dad in the hallway. Her name's Kari. She's not doing well. She has *B. cepacia*."

C3, the unit I was staying in, is often called the CF ghetto because it gets a steady flow of us. Sometimes, in the winter months, we flood C3 in waves, but even in summer there are always at least a few of us. We're hard to miss, especially if you know what to look for: skinny arms and legs that seem too small for the rest of the body, rattling cough, white mesh sleeve covering a PICC line, four daily visits from RTs, an IV pole with many lines coming from it. Even though we recognize each other, there isn't a protocol for the first approach. Patient confidentiality trumps the need for social connection.

I watched Kari and her dad as they walked along the perimeter of the hospital, focusing on the eerily skinny shadow cast by her legs. When I'm well enough my mom and I sneak off the hospital grounds to go for longer walks to the Stanford Shopping Center, and I suspected that's what they were doing. I found myself curious: What was her situation? How sick was she? Was she able to go to college? Was she happy?

The next morning, I learned that Kari's dad and my mom had seen each other in the hallway and had bonded over our shared life experience. They arranged for us to meet, so the next day we met at the fountain.

One of the great tragedies of CF is that in addition to isolating patients from healthy peers, it also isolates patients from each other. Cross-infection, or transmission of a bacterial infection from one patient to another, is one of the most serious concerns in the CF community. Physical interaction with other patients can be extremely dangerous, so it's highly discouraged. Patients are segregated from each other as a matter of course; we are not allowed to touch, stand within fifteen feet of each other, or be in each other's vicinity without a mask on. For those of us with *B. cepacia*—only about 3 percent of patients—patient contact is expressly forbidden; in the small print at the bottom of any invitation, website, or brochure regarding any CF event read the words, "No patient with a positive culture for *B. cepacia* complex may attend."

I'd never actually met anyone with CF in person before coming to Stanford and was happy to meet up with Kari the next day as she walked out of the hospital holding her dad for support. We exchanged small talk for a few minutes, both struggling to know what to say before talking about the things we so desperately wanted to discuss.

"Where are you from?" I asked.

"I live in Oregon but I've been coming to Stanford for the CF clinic since I had my liver transplant at fourteen," she began. She spoke more quietly than I did and was much smaller; even though she's two years older, she looks at least five years younger than me. "I used to go to OSU, but now I take classes online so I can live at home. My brother's just starting there as a freshman. We're both so excited . . . him to start college, and me because I get to retain my link to OSU."

I told her that I go to Stanford, that I'm a junior, that I live in and staff a freshman dorm. Then I didn't know how to proceed. I had been so excited to meet her but when the moment came, my true questions evaporated and my brain emptied. We were silent for a bit, but I wasn't uncomfortable, and she didn't appear to be, either. She struck me as stoic and thoughtful. A strong fighter, but very much at peace. Radiant smile lighting up a beautiful face atop a frail body. Finally, we started talking about what was going on with her health in this current hospitalization.

"This week has been challenging," she admitted. "Because my lung function is so low now, I was evaluated for a double-lung transplant. But I was denied."

My heart sank. When CF patients get to a certain point in the progression of the disease, the last remaining option for saving their lives is a double-lung transplant. New lungs often mean a second chance at life for people who would otherwise soon die. Any patient near end-stage disease hopes they will be strong enough to be eligible for transplant.

"Because of my *B. cepacia,* my previous liver transplant, and my weight, they said I wouldn't survive the transplant," she announced evenly. "So they won't do it."

"But . . . but . . . is that it?" I sputtered. "They won't change their minds? What's going to happen?"

"The doctor told me he wished he could give me some hope, but there was nothing they could do. 'We're going to help you live your life as long as these lungs will allow, but eventually you will be looking at hospice,' he said to me. 'Is that a term you're familiar with?' It was so abrupt. I was reactionless." My eyes were fixed on her as she told me this, but she was looking down at the water. She paused for a moment, opened her mouth to continue, but then hesitated.

"Are . . . are you okay?" I asked. It wasn't the right thing to say, but nothing was. I wanted to give her a hug so badly, not just for her but for myself as well.

She looked up and this time looked me right in the eye. "All I could think about was how my best friend asked me recently what I was most looking forward to after my transplant. I said I was so excited to be able to laugh again. I can't now; my lungs are too weak and it hurts. I was really looking forward to that, to getting my laugh back."

My body stiffened. I was heartbroken for her and stunned

that she was so calm after hearing the worst piece of news a CF patient could hear. But I didn't want to pry.

"When did this happen?" I finally allowed.

"Yesterday."

We both fell silent again for a while. I curled my toes in the water and tried to focus on how the sun felt on the nape of my neck, hoping to shut out the questions I was dying to ask.

"Don't you just wish sometimes your life could be like a Taylor Swift song?" she asked, smiling a little bitterly. I nodded in grim agreement.

A few days later, I was discharged from the hospital and moved back into my dorm room. Kari had to stay a while longer.

As I got to know Kari, I learned more about her situation. The way I see it, all CF patients live on a continuum somewhere between the health of birth and the impending death from end-stage disease. How fast one moves along that continuum differs from person to person, and how much control we have over that is debated. Kari's a bit farther along than I am, and so is another CF-er I've met, Caleigh.

A year ago, during an inpatient stay at Stanford Hospital, a rattling cough echoing through the wall between my room and the one next door signaled to me that the patient was one of my people. On daily walks through the halls, I slowed down in front of her doorway to peek inside, wanting to put a face to the cough. When she walked by my room, I saw her do the same.

On my fourth day in-house, during CPT, I asked my RT if the girl next door had CF. He said yes but would not tell me her name. "I'd get fired for breaking every patient privacy policy in existence." But an hour after he left my room, he came back holding a slip of paper. "Don't tell anyone," he whispered nervously, "but she wanted to meet you, too." An untidy scrawl on the paper read: *"Caleigh Haber. Add me on Facebook. I'd love to talk!"* Five minutes later, we were chatting online. Like prison inmates who communicate by knocking on connecting walls, we spent our days twenty feet apart, getting acquainted through the computer without hearing each other's voices.

About a week later, my dad and I were roaming the halls to get exercise. Rounding a corner, I saw a little girl walking ahead with her back to me. She looked no more than eighty pounds and pulled an IV pole alongside her. A small dog walked beside her and there was a woman, too. We kept our distance, not wanting to intrude. When they reached the end of the hall, they turned around and started to walk back, and that's when I realized that this wasn't a child. It was my neighbor.

"Caleigh!" I called out, loud enough for her to hear but quiet enough not to disturb patients nearby. "It's Mallory!" We sat down in the hall, separated by masks and fifteen feet of space to avoid cross-infection, and finally talked face to-face. She was very frank. She told me how her life had diverged completely from the lives of her friends and how, in her opinion, peer alienation was the worst part of CF.

"It's a constant struggle to get out of bed in the morning," she told me. "To eat the calories I need to gain weight despite constant stomach pain, to spend four or more hours a day doing my breathing treatments, to fight fatigue, to sterilize, cook, clean, exercise, and sleep, but most of all, to be in such close proximity to the life I want but can never have."

Throughout our conversation, we marveled at the parallels between our lives. Caleigh was twenty-one. I was nineteen. Caleigh had been a cheerleader in high school. I played volleyball and swam. We were both from Southern California and relocated to NorCal for college, both had been active and outgoing in high school, both had enjoyed relatively stable lung function throughout high school, which had allowed us to feel somewhat normal when we weren't in the hospital. At the time of our meeting, I was a sophomore in college; she had just finished culinary school and was working as a chef.

In her four years since high school, Caleigh's lung function had declined from 70 percent to less than 30 percent. In my two years since high school, my lung function had declined from 70 percent to 50 percent. Her story made my heart sink; although it was comforting to see the parallels between our lives and to be able to talk about them, it was also a reminder of how much scarier my disease could become and how quickly that could happen. We had been pursuing our dreams with the same tenacity, suffering similar accelerating disease progression as a result.

Caleigh's story of rapid lung function decline seemed like a manifest warning, a road sign reminding me to slow down to avoid careening off a cliff. Two years ago, Caleigh was at that fateful curve; now, in free fall, her lung function was at 18 percent, and her lungs had been colonized by MRSA (methicillin-resistant *Staphylococcus aureus,* a species of bacteria almost as virulent as *B. cepacia*). Because of her low body weight, she, too, had been denied a transplant. I'm not sure she had the benefit of warning signs, the signs in my life that were Kari and Caleigh. Their stories forced me to question the way I live.

Kari, Caleigh, and I have a deep unspoken connection, forged in the halls and courtyards of Stanford Hospital. After meeting both of them, I connected them online; they now provide each other with a lot of support. We're an unusual "trio," the two of them so small that a slight breeze could knock them over, and me standing at six feet. Kari has an unwavering faith in God and radiates compassion with quiet courage and resilience. Caleigh has boundless energy kept in check only by her diminished lung function. Caleigh's spirited irreverence fuels a fearless commitment to surpassing expectations. And then there's me, the one who never actually *looks* sick. A few years behind the other two in progression and age, closer to Caleigh in beliefs but to Kari in disposition, seemingly so lucky by comparison, even though their reality will ultimately be mine. I'm at a loss for how to comfort them.

Their lives leave me with profound questions about my own future. If we're all straddling that line between the real world and the war world of chronic illness, they spend much more time on the battlefront and get to feel normalcy much less frequently. Maybe where I am is actually the training camp, and they've already been deployed. When I think about how many years they have left, it's hard not to think of them as future versions of myself, and fear that my prognosis will soon be as bleak as theirs. With a deep breath, I remind myself that they are not actually warning messengers. Each patient has her own progression. My disease has proven itself to be a cunning and unpredictable enemy, attacking from the inside like a Trojan horse. But even as this battle rages, even as every decision becomes more significant and every complication more ominous, the real world continues, providing one day after the next, each good day unfolding as a fleeting, beautiful gift.

I have the feeling that there's nothing *after* this, that this life is all we're ever going to get, and it's fragile and brief and easier to throw away than we think. This understanding drives the way I carry myself from the time I open my eyes in the morning to when I close them in sleep. When I lie in bed at night, I think about mortality, about what I want. I hope that what I want is realistic . . . but fear that it's not.

A few weeks ago, I went back to C3 to stop by Caleigh's room. My few weeks out of the hospital had been a refreshing break, but I felt a strange sense of relief and belonging when I walked back into clinic and up to C3. I'd spoken to Caleigh many times in the past couple of months, since she'd been in the hospital for a very long time.

I'd gone to the market and picked up chocolate, cheese, crackers, berries, and magazines, all the while wearing gloves so I wouldn't touch any of it. I asked her nurse to give Caleigh my care package: Caleigh was delighted by the gift but she couldn't eat any of it because she was having surgery the next day. I chatted with her for a few minutes from the doorway. She was less animated than usual. Her mom told me in private that a release date was nowhere in sight. Putting on my best smile, I filled her in on my life but kept it very brief; I know how hard it is to hear the details of others' "normal lives" out in the real world when you're entrenched as an inpatient. When I told her a funny story about my first volleyball practice, she laughed and immediately started coughing, cringing in pain; this made me think of Kari, and I wondered how she was doing.

It was time for me to go, but saying goodbye was hard. I waved and said, "See you soon," then slowly walked down the long hallway. I was grateful to be able to leave, but my gratitude was tempered by the awareness that they could not. And I, with the freedom of a soaring bird—if not forever, then at least in that moment—escaped to the real world, while they, like birds with broken wings, lay bedridden.

2014

1/10/14
I'm still pissed that Stanford won't let me go back on ataluren, so I sent this:

To the Research Team:

I started ataluren the summer before my freshman year of
college, sometime between June and August 2010. In the
spring of 2010, before the trial, I lost 13 pounds, was in the
hospital for 4 weeks receiving 3 antibiotics and IV lipids, and
suffered an episode of life-threatening sepsis. I continued IVs
for a total of 12 weeks. Despite receiving 2,000 calories a
day of IV lipids I could not gain weight, and after 12 weeks
on IVs my lung function did not improve.

When I started taking ataluren, I thought the best I
could hope for would be to stay stable. It didn't cross my
mind that my lung function would get better, as that's not
typically how my disease progression has worked in the
past. Once my baseline drops it tends to stay down and
not rise back up. But within just a few months, I was
gaining weight and my lung function was increasing
despite living a less healthy lifestyle than I ever had in the
past (exercising less, skipping more treatments, sleeping
less, college drinking, etc.). Every other year of college
since then, one or two skipped treatments, one night of
bad sleep, or a few days without exercise could cause an
exacerbation and land me in the hospital. But in that year
and the summer following (when I was on ataluren), it
seemed that nothing I did could really make me sick.

Yes, I do know that I got sick in the fall of my sophomore year, when I was still on ataluren. However, there
were significant changes that occurred that I believe are
responsible for that first exacerbation in 16 months. I
became a vegetarian that summer, and being a vegetarian
with other dietary restrictions and eating in a dining hall
meant I started to lose weight. I lived in a triple room with

roommates who did not understand how important cleanliness was to my well-being; the room was deemed by the school to be a bio-safety hazard because it was moldy and filled with germs. I spent three weeks before school started in an intensive arts program where I did not have adequate time to do treatment, sleep, or exercise. I had no help moving into my room, didn't have time to unpack for weeks, and couldn't find some of my medications. I only slept about five or six hours a night those first few months because of my increased academic load and class schedule. My mental state was not ideal because I was extremely stressed about school and the living/eating situation.

All of these things preceded that first exacerbation. It makes no sense to me to attribute the exacerbation to ataluren. I was going to need a hospitalization eventually, and with all of those issues that fall of 2011, not even ataluren could protect me. But I got much worse after I stopped taking ataluren that year. Once I stopped the drug I developed a pulmonary embolism, elevated liver enzymes, gallstones, a fungal cavitation, etc., and lost all the weight I had gained the previous year. I do not think I would have declined so much or had so many complications my sophomore year or after that had I been on ataluren.

I am aware of the placebo effect and the fact that regular doctor visits as part of a clinical trial can have a beneficial effect whether you're on the study drug or not. But I have always had regular doctor visits, both before and after enrolling at Stanford. This is something my parents insisted on, and when I was treated at Cedars-Sinai, I was free to just "pop in" whenever I felt the slightest symptom. As the patient, the person who experienced both the benefit of the first 16 months and the harm that ensued, I believe with 100% certainty that the drug made a huge difference in my quality of life and I want that back. I've lost so much lung function in the past three years that my life is barely recognizable, and I see the possibilities in my future shrinking. I don't think it's fair to exclude a patient from a trial this life-changing because of one pulmonary exacerbation that was BOUND to happen with or without the drug.

On a more philosophical level, this flat-out rejection dashes my hopes of ever getting a lung transplant. I know that my case is complicated on paper. But every doctor has said my clinical presentation doesn't match what they see in the chart. If trials and transplant teams and doctors never took on complicated patients, it would do a great disservice to the CF community.

Let's talk about the specific yellow and red flags you mentioned.

1. Aminoglycoside usage—I would be happy to commit to not taking TOBI* in any form. I never really thought TOBI worked for me. Ataluren is much more important to me.

2. Stability—how long do I have to be out of the hospital to qualify? All CF patients have exacerbations, and the one I had in December was extremely minor. I was in the hospital only 5 days. I don't see why this is grounds for exclusion.

3. Recent anticoagulation—one doctor called my pulmonary embolism "subclinical," and said it was discovered only by accident through a CT scan. He thought it

---

* an effective antibiotic that is taken through a nebulizer

didn't warrant any treatment at all. Another doctor did think it warranted anticoagulants, which I did for 3 months. The risk factor I had for a clotting disorder was birth control pills. I have since discontinued oral birth control . . . so there's no reason why I should need anticoagulants again.

4. GI issues—doesn't every CF patient have GI issues?
5. *B. cepacia*—I had *B. cepacia* when I started the trial last time and it wasn't grounds for exclusion then.
6. Hemoptysis—same as answer for *"B. cepacia."*
7. Fungal lung infection—are you referring to the fungal infection I had in 2011? Or current cultures for fungi? As far as I know, I have 7 colonies of fungus, which the clinic assured me are minor and don't warrant treatment.

I hope you understand why I think being on ataluren would change the trajectory of my life. Please let me know what you think.

The answer was nonresponsive.

2/9/14

I've been working out every day and feeling pretty strong—and my lungs feel pretty good! Feels like a miracle.

I've started reading this book called *How to Be Sick,* a Buddhist-inspired guide to living well with chronic illness and being happy. Which sounds super cheesy and stupid, but I feel like the author shares a lot of similarities with me. A lot of what the author describes, I'm like yes, yes, yes and find myself wanting to underline it and highlight stuff. I think part of it is coming to accept your fate and accept that discomfort, disease, struggle, and hardship are part of life. To not fight against your situation or try to change it.

To accept that what you have is not going to go away and to learn how to live well anyway.

Part of me bristles against this because it feels like it's like giving up. The author explains it's not giving up, but rather giving in to the possibility that your life will constantly evolve and change in ways you never predicted, and it's important to be able to live happily with disease instead of waiting to be healthy before being satisfied and happy with life. I do agree with that.

Sometimes I'm at peace with my reality . . . but sometimes I feel as if there's something inside me that's shaking and wobbly and anxious and scared. Something I can't describe that makes it feel like things are *not* right. But I'm hoping that as I read this book and try to incorporate that mentality into my life, I will feel at peace and truly grateful for what I have, and optimistic, not necessarily about the length of my life or my health status, but about what I can do even if my health isn't great.

I want to live in a state of serenity and happiness that's *stable,* not ephemeral and dependent on outside circumstances. That's the goal. Hopefully *How to Be Sick* will help, and I think it will because I'm in chapter 2 and it's already spurred this reflection.

The coed bathroom situation just doesn't work for me, and it's weird because it's not like I'm into any of the guys in this dorm, so I don't know why it matters, but this is just always an issue for me. Public bathrooms are fine but only when they're single sex. My stomach seems to be the thing that puts me in the worst mood . . . lung problems just don't.

Another stress—the pitch I have to write for my CF/environment podcast that Julie Snyder of *This American Life* will read is due at 6:00 p.m. tomorrow. And Jonah* is SO strict on deadlines, and I haven't started it and I'm probably not going to get back

* the manager of the Stanford Storytelling Project

until 4:30 and when I do get back I will have only slept like four to five hours probably. Ugh. But I'm not going to let it get to me. I'll finish it and it will turn out fine. It isn't every day you get the chance to get your work read by NPR. Stanford provides amazing opportunities!

4/1/14

Gotta love class assignments cuz they force me to remember and to write:

The sea turtle (the honu) is a sacred animal, an ancient Hawaiian symbol for longevity, safety, emotional strength, and wisdom. Hawaiian legend has it that the honu guided Polynesians to the islands, so many Hawaiians revere the honu as a guardian spirit, an aumakua, which protects them. They evolved long before dinosaurs went extinct and long before the Hawaiian Islands were even formed.

It was 2012 in Maui, my sophomore year of college. My lung function was 50 percent. For the past year, I'd been slammed with complication after complication, and I'd been in the hospital five times. It seemed like every organ system of my body had suffered abuse. I was in a really dark place, and for the first time, I was diagnosed with depression.

One day, in the middle of the trip, I woke up and everything felt heavy—my body, my head, my heart. Driving to the beach, I had a hard time looking at the sun—the day was too bright, the sky too blue. When I got there, I went straight for the ocean and dove in, trying to hold my breath as long as I could so I could stay there, because it was the only place where the pieces of myself came close to coming back together again. I was thinking about mortality and disease progression and acceleration. And I felt helpless and vulnerable and broken.

I started to cry underwater and the salty tears were mingling with the salt water of the ocean. And I was completely alone. But then I wasn't. I had exhaled all of my breath, so I could sink down below the surface a bit and I was lying faceup, looking at the sky through the water, and all of a sudden, something appeared in my right field of vision. This honu, this green sea turtle, swam up, and it got really close to me and just sort of stopped and hung there and stayed close. And I was probably imagining this, but it felt like it was looking at me, not just looking at me but really seeing me. And I looked back at this creature, with its brown shell and cracked skin and large dark eyes, and thought to myself that it had come along at that moment for a reason. I'm not a spiritual person, but I had an epiphany that that one sea turtle helped set me on the path to feeling whole again.

I still struggled for a long time after that, but I will never forget that moment, looking at that turtle and imagining that it was looking back with compassion. My soul felt endangered at the time by the threats to my body, and that turtle made me feel as if I did have the strength to ride through the turbulence of my disease with grace. Eventually, I had a resurgence of hope, and I realized that my future would hold a lot more happiness and promise than I allowed myself to believe.

My depression was a critical turning point in my battle with cystic fibrosis. I really thought my future would be one of continual decline and then death from respiratory failure or organ rejection of transplanted lungs.

Even though I descended into a deep depression for parts of my sophomore year of college, even though I live today in objectively worse health standing than ever with a lung function of about 40 percent, I've never felt more hopeful, more resilient, more empowered. I'm fighting for the future health of my body.

I didn't ask for illness but I own it, because if I don't, no one else will. And taking ownership has empowered me to believe that things can change.

4/4/14

I'm insanely worried about my friend Melissa. She has CF, took
a deep dive, and went technology-MIA for weeks because she
was so sick. She's on 20 liters of O$_2$. I'm on TWO. She finally
got in touch and sent me a video tonight. She's having severe
anxiety and PTSD about being back in the hospital, under-
standably. I can't even think about it without crying. She seemed
so dejected in the video, maybe sedated, and so weary. Just about
how I feel, but she has a better excuse.

5/10/14

When I was nine, I decided to stop doing my breathing treatments. They took too long. None of my friends had to do them.
I was sick of being different when I felt and looked just like
other kids. My mother tried pleading, bribing, punishing, and
yelling, but without success. My dad came home early from
work to talk to me. I avoided his gaze as we sat facing each other
across the kitchen table.

"Mallory," he said, "your mother and I do not ask you to do
your treatments so you'll feel better. We do not ask you to do
them so you won't get sick." He paused. "We ask you to do them
so you won't die. If you don't do your treatments, *you will die.*"

I burst into tears, leapt up from the table, and ran to my room,
slamming the door behind me. I hated them. I hated that keeping
myself alive was such an inconvenience, I hated that my dad forced
me to face my own mortality, and I hated that they were right.
For three days, I didn't speak to my parents. But since that day,
I've never refused treatment, because I know what's at stake. It's
not a matter of preference or convenience; it's a matter of life or
death.

I asked my dad recently about that day. Did he have to resort to such extreme measures to get me to comply? "Sometimes," he said, "tough love and brutal honesty are the only arrows left in our quiver."

That conversation twelve years ago made me realize that we cannot possess true emotional maturity without a deep awareness of the stakes of our actions. At age nine, the consequences of my choices were too far away for me to consider; someone had to shove reality in my face for me to realize what I was risking.

Humanity is living like seven billion nine-year-olds. We don't accept that what we do now will hurt us later. The disparity between my seriousness and others' flippancy regarding the planet drives me to use my experience facing illness and mortality to force people's eyes open, so they have no choice but to understand what's at stake.

Ever since my parents threw me into the water at age three, the ocean has been my escape, my passion, and a powerful healing agent. I've always faced complications of cystic fibrosis, from malnutrition to frequent and aggressive pneumonias. For years, I've had the unshakable sense that being in nature (and specifically, the ocean) somehow heals me. Clears my lungs. Prolongs my life. Maintains my sanity. Restores my soul.

My intuition was right. While I was swimming, surfing, and fighting CF, researchers in Australia were discovering what I already knew: CF patients who frequent the ocean live longer—ten years longer.

The concepts of sustainability and human health are intertwined. The sustainability of the planet is the cornerstone of human health. Every person, whether they accept it or not, depends on this planet for survival: air, water, and food. But we have adopted a paradigm that separates humans from the rest of nature. Though we owe our existence to the planet, most of us are passive

bystanders, watching idly as development and destruction demol-
ish our temple. We assume Earth will keep on giving, no matter
what.

My health fluctuates more than a healthy person's, so I'm
acutely aware how my health declines in sick environments. In a
polluted city, I cough, wheeze, and breathe with pain. Ocean
swimming, the most effective natural therapy, harms me when the
water is dirty. Simultaneously learning about environmental destruction and coping with the rapid progression of my disease, I
was struck by parallels between my own struggling body and the
planet itself.

As CF progresses, mucus builds up in my lungs, harboring
bacteria and inviting an immune response that erodes the gas-
exchange tissue. I push my body to function, but my destiny is
dictated by my DNA.

The planet is diseased, too, and like any other organism
would, it's crying out for help. The visible signs of environmental
destruction are outnumbered by the invisible ones, just like the
damage inflicted by cystic fibrosis. But while I can talk about my
disease, garnering sympathy and support, the environment can't.

Human sickness and environmental destruction are one and
the same. The bacteria in my lungs are to me what the human
species is to the planet. It's just a matter of scale and perspective.
My experiences make me want to shake people and scream, "This
is what it feels like! If we don't do something, this is what will
happen."

6/15/14
Today I graduated college (well . . . I walked). It was a beautiful
day. Beautiful ceremony. For Wacky Walk, a Stanford tradition,
I was a tree with Maya, while Gia and Danny were tree huggers.
I thought I would be too exhausted to enjoy the festivities, but

it was too big of a day with too much adrenaline not to. The ceremony was NOT boring; Bill and Melinda Gates gave a great speech.

The day started in the Stanford stadium with the entire class (before we split off for our department graduations). I feel lucky to be in such a beautiful place with amazing intellectual and social vitality. And to be healthy enough to be part of the celebration. It's a miracle that I wasn't hospitalized my entire last quarter at Stanford! I'm so incredibly grateful!

One thing that dampened the joy was news that a senior was found dead in his dorm room—they think by suicide. Xavier and I lived in the same dorm sophomore year—Toyon. It's unfathomable to think about. Devastating. On graduation day. The worst part is that he went to Wacky Walk this morning and then back to his room to kill himself. His sister went to find him when he didn't show up to his department ceremony. My heart breaks for him and his family.

6/27/14

Home! At first glance, I saw that everything was as it had always been. The olive tree in the front yard hung over neglected grass, making an obnoxious show of its vitality. The warmth of the house—in both color and temperature—enveloped me, setting off powerful pangs of nostalgia. Even the smell of coffee, extra dark roast, brought me back to adolescence, to early mornings and big breakfasts before school.

In my room, I sat on the bed. Here, things were different— I couldn't decide if my quarters, with their newly white walls, white dresser, and dark wood floors, looked elegant or sterile. Part of me missed the messy oranges, pinks, and greens of my childhood bedroom. One photo of me with friends, propped up on the dresser in a cheap, plastic frame, had survived the great "clutter purge" that my mom had undertaken. It was from an old disposable camera, the kind no one used anymore. It was grainy, but the happiness on the faces of my best friends was unmistakable.

Other things were different, too, I realized. No white-coated lanky Labrador had bounded up to the window by the front door to see my face before greeting me. Since Dewey died, the house felt a little bit emptier. The fridge was emptier, too, the pantry barren in support of my dad's low-fat, low-calorie, low-sodium diet. My mom offered to whip up a protein smoothie and a chicken stir-fry for me in support of the high-fat, high-calorie, high-sodium diet my doctors wanted. I declined, feeling more overwhelmed than underfed.

At the entrance to my room, I stood and looked down the long hallway to the front door. Our house has a terribly closed-off floor plan, not good for the entertaining my mom so loved to do; but she always made it work anyway. I loved this house that I'd grown up in. But on this day, the day I came home to L.A. after graduating, that narrow hallway was a stifling physical reminder of my narrowing prospects. I shouldn't have been home—not to stay, at least. My pride, nostalgia, ambition, confusion, fear, and fatigue all mingled together as if gurgling in a cauldron.

7/15/14

So happy to be spending the summer in Hawaii. Becca and Ari didn't come when I did so in the beginning my mom stayed with me and then Jesse, Gaby, Ali, and Stacy visited!

Fourth of July here was crazy. They have this annual event called Floatilla!!!! A tangle of hippies, drunks, military folks, surfers, tourists—hanging out in the water on a formation of floats! Loud music coming through speakers, phones submerged in plastic cases, alcohol being passed around freely like it was water. Fireball bottles floating in the water. Recycling bins on paddle-boards, good Samaritans collecting beer bottles. Pacific Drunk-People-on-Rafts Patch is the new Pacific Garbage Patch. You have to Jet Ski to get out there; it can barely be seen from shore. I went with Gaby and Stacy but we got separated in the crowd. So much fun but ended up with fever so had to cut it short. A kindhearted man paddled me back. In a crazy turn of events, Stacy ended up dating him.

10/10/14

What an incredible summer in Hawaii. After the Fourth, it was so busy, so fun, I didn't need to write. But thinking back I marvel at the prowess of my body and how incredible those three months were. Documenting to remember:

6:00 a.m. surf sessions in glassy conditions. Paddling for hours, never getting cold, never getting tired. Pop-up after pop-up, wave after wave. Infatuation with Shawn, my friend . . . my surf guru . . . my what-even-are-you?

Confusion, mixed signals, so much laughter.

One day, coughing up blood before a surf date, I considered canceling and decided against it, too excited to see him, too worried that if I canceled, I'd never surf with him again. As unpredictable as he was at the beginning of the summer, just out of my grasp, is how consistent he later became, dependable, loving, and ever-there.

Papayas and frozen waffles, açai bowls and coffee. Sustenance that fueled my surf habit. The daily drive along that road from Kahala to Waikiki, from the suburbs to the surf in our sturdy Toyota 4Runner rental. Boards hanging out the hatchback, "Take Me to Church," by Hozier, blaring from the speakers.

Sandy feet on my yoga mat, the sweet teacher we'd see after

class at Whole Foods. Our bodies would sweat salt onto the salt already on our skin from the surf beforehand.

Surfing with DJ one day in front of the Kaimana cottage. Disorganized surf spot with shifty surf, lots of reef. Trying to escape the crowds, we paddled way out to a break where only very advanced surfers were lining up. We planned to stay on the inside and catch the smaller ones, staying out of the way of the others. My arms got tired on my seven-foot, six-inch Sippy Noserider so I switched boards with him, taking his eleven-foot log, heavy as lead.

A six-footer rolled through and I noticed too late to paddle over it; the wave tossed me off the board and the massive fin sliced half the circumference of my thigh just above the knee, then down the back of the leg to the mid-calf. Didn't break skin, thank God, but caused a hematoma the size of a softball. The pain it caused left me immobile for weeks.

Tandem surfing competition with Shawn in Duke's Oceanfest. Learning how to do lifts with Bear, the World Tandem Surfing Champion. Shawn's magnetic smile, his mind-boggling ability to surf while holding me in the air.

Pali Highway, surrounded by towering heights of green, like the set of *Jurassic Park*. That time it rained down on us when we were in an open Jeep, when it went from sunny skies to pouring buckets in an instant.

Windy days on those beautiful east side beaches, Kailua, Lanikai. The Whole Foods in Kailua where they jacked up the price of water when Hurricanes Julio and Iselle were coming. The hurricanes were supposed to devastate the island; we prepared to be indoors for days, bought hundreds of dollars of water. Safeway stores all over the island were out of water. We hunkered down; the Big Island was ravaged.

My roommates, my partners in crime, my incredible friends.

Becca and Ari, BFFs for life. Other friendships forged. And Shawn. Always Shawn. One day I found out my unrequited feelings turned out not to be unrequited. Double-date night on Taco Tuesday, alcohol and greasy tortilla chips and then, sadly, fevers.

Mom flying in to help me move home. The very last night, massive hemoptysis and hospitalization the next day. Shawn showing up with fresh-picked avocados from the mountain, sunflowers, and dominoes. Yoga and sneaking out to secret patios. Dr. Mohabir saying I couldn't fly home. Ten days in the hospital followed by a ten-day hotel stay since our lease was up.

Those three weeks of sickness when everything changed, with us, and with my health.

That summer of 2014 was freedom. It was fantasy. My life was a movie that I didn't want to end. No perception of my body being limited in any way until my very last night on the island. Every day, I did what I wanted and my body obliged. It supported my purest passions and athletic endeavors.

That summer we did the ledge. I stood on the highest tower, seeing the most beautiful world in every direction. And then hemoptysis. I plunged, free-fall. The fabric of my perfect life unraveled.

Now I see no rock-holds or crevices to help me climb. There is no climbing back up. When you're falling, there's only one direction you can go.

10/15/14

I made a big decision yesterday—I talked with my professor Andrew Todhunter for about an hour. Told him about my options for work post Stanford and how I was feeling lost and confused about what I should do. He advised me to avoid a real job (important to hear from an adult who's not one of my parents). I know they want me to avoid a real job for health reasons, and Andrew has the perspective of a healthy person who avoided a real job for different reasons.

Andrew encouraged me to become a writer and to take on a book project (to write about Susan Gottlieb, an important environmentalist, and her renowned native garden). Reasons:

- I care deeply about the environment
- Will make money
- Great on my résumé
- Give me confidence to do a book-length project
- Experience will translate when I'm ready to write my own book.

I talked to Andrew about what's important to me, and how to go about being a writer. What the days are like, how to keep yourself on track/disciplined, how to network to get work. Lots of philosophical talk, but also lots of practical talk. He's so helpful. Later met with James Campbell (another one of my professors), who is so inspiring.

10/16/14
When I was young, I learned about the selfish gene.

Lying in bed at night, cuddled beneath the covers, my dad's voice would soothe me to sleep with talk about the complexity of the human genome, the spiral shape of a DNA helix, the way forces of natural selection would make harmful mutations die out with their host, but allow random beneficial mutations to proliferate and spread through a population, causing such changes within a species that one common ancestor could play grandfather to a bonobo, a rhesus monkey, and a human, or a Brussels sprout, mustard seed, and stalk of broccoli.

Every night, as he'd wax poetic about the marvels of evolutionary biology, only taking a break to throw in some astrophysics and history, I'd fall asleep to the letters A, T, C, and G, amazed at this world we live in, developing this *profound love* for the theory of evolution, for the belief that random chance and probability could shape a planet composed of rock, water, and protozoa into the beautifully varied community of life that exists today, from the highest peaks of the Himalayas to the lush richness of the Amazon to the eerie black depths of the dark ocean floor.

We worshipped Dawkins and Dennett, the unusual versions of childhood heroes my brother and I clung to, and they illuminated if not the why, then at least the how of human existence. Evolution seemed like a religion, but it wasn't one because it does not require faith, it encourages you to question, to dig, literally, to understand the origin of our species and the complex history of the genetic matter that existed, mutated, and evolved to construct this current world of ours. This community of species we share the planet with, a community that has lost members like the dodo, the Kauai o'o bird, the Caribbean monk seal, the Baiji white dolphin.

We read *God's Debris* and *The God Delusion*, debunked the logical proof of God's existence put forth by Aquinas, read the Bible as literature, and occasionally laughed at the more outland-ish elements of certain stories—Lot's wife turning to a pillar of salt for looking over her shoulder, Joseph's brothers' inability to rec-ognize him when he became pharaoh of Egypt, Noah's Ark and the idea that two of every species alive today could fit into one boat without all eating each other, the blood in the river and the frogs and the leeches; but we learned some lessons anyway, in Sunday school and in discussions at the dinner table, what my parents called the "point" of their atheist version of Judaism.

But one day, I realized that evolution, the almighty natural force that I revered with the core of my being . . . *evolution isn't acting on me.*

I'm exempt.

If natural selection were happening unhindered, I would be dead. There would be no Mallory Smith, age twenty-two, Stanford graduate living and breathing, making friends and reflecting on the origins of the universe. There would just be some ashes scattered in the Pacific Ocean, or however my family would choose to honor a life that had no chance to ripen.

I was born with two defective copies of the CFTR gene,* one mutated copy from each parent. You have one copy of the gene, and you get a heterozygote advantage, an increased fitness because of a lower likelihood of dying of cholera. But with two copies of the gene, you're salty. The old adage goes, "The child will soon die whose brow tastes salty when kissed."

At this point, keeping myself alive is a full-fledged mission, enlisting all of my energy and hours of my day, every day, as I need nine to ten hours of sleep, sixteen pills with a hearty breakfast, packing extra calories to overcome malnutrition caused by pancreatic insufficiency. Vitamins and minerals, probiotics and antibiotics, gastrointestinal medications, sinus rinses with saline, steroids and antibiotics, lengthy CPT treatments. All to reduce inflammation and fight the chronic deadly infection eating away at my fragile, scarred lungs.

And that's just the morning.

Throughout the day, more pills four times a day. Some three times a day, some every time I eat, some thirty minutes before eating. Another round of CPT/vest midday, more breathing treatments. Then the entire morning routine again at night.

About four hours a day I dedicate to the simple act of taking a breath, fighting the billions of bacteria overtaking my lungs and clearing out the mucus so I don't feel like I'm breathing through

* cystic fibrosis transmembrane conductance regulator gene

a straw with a boulder weighing on my chest. Staying alive, for someone with CF, requires active and constant effort *against* natural selection, requires a grand *fuck you* to that force which, left to its own devices, would have us suffocated from respiratory failure before adolescence.

What does my survival come down to, what is responsible for my ability to trump natural selection? Medicine. Medicine gives me the gift of life. Medicine exempts me from the forces that paved the way for humanity to emerge, that shaped life on Earth for millions of years, since the very first cell sprung to life in the primordial soup.

How is that fair? Why do we, today, get to override evolution? What will that do for the future of our species? More important, what does that mean for the millions of other species on this planet who don't have that unfair advantage, who still exist at evolution's mercy?

I want to live and I want people the world over affected with illness, ridden with deadly diseases, to live, to survive, to *thrive*, and to reproduce, creating imperfect little perfects. I want us to be viewed as worthy enough to pass on our genes, even if we'd be outcompeted by those whose genome is "better" in a world where natural selection still reigned supreme.

My life is a miracle. Life in general is a miracle. Our existence is the result of stars exploding, solar systems forming, our Earth having an environment hospitable to life, and then, finally, millions of highly improbable events accumulating over millions of years to bring us, a capable and conscious bag of stardust, to the here and now.

PART THREE

Mallory had the craziest nicknames for people. For example, Talia was Takau, Gaby was Gikatu, Maya was Mizzle or Missoula Humes, Mark and Micah were Pidge and Bridge. We'd always crack up about what she'd come up with. As for my nickname, Mal called me Alsballs so I called her Mallzballs, which over time became just Balls. I was the left ball, she was the right ball. Despite Mal's genius, she was playful and silly and sometimes downright goofy. There are so many funny and irreverent stories to tell about my best friend.

—ALISON EPSTEIN

2015

2/1/15

The last time I wrote was a few days after my birthday. That shouldn't bug me. I was happy, I was busy, I didn't write, who cares? I actually do care. Because there were a lot of times I felt like I needed to write to clarify things in my life, and I didn't, because I hadn't written recently and I wasn't in a mood at that particular moment to catch my own journal up on my own life. Deep regrets.

2/10/15

Life is good.

Spent a week up at Stanford for medical appointments, seeing college friends plus Talia and Jason in the city. Spent time on campus, working and walking around, soaking in the beauty, and it was really nice. Felt good enough to go to yoga and play beach volleyball twice!

Then came home to L.A., spent one day here recovering and sleeping, then dove into Susan's book. Flew to Vegas with Natasha's friends. Stayed in a villa at the Mirage—a villa that normally costs $11,000 a night but Sasha's dad got as a favor because he did eye surgery on someone important. It looked like Versailles.

The day was so much fun. By the time we walked to the club I was tipsy. We had a private table and were being waited on like kings. We danced, then I sat down because I started to cough. Natasha went with me to the bathroom so I could cough up mucus (alcohol thins mucus and so does laughing). The attendant thought my violent coughing was barfing. And my nose was oozing blood (an ongoing problem of late, plus it's dry in the desert and alcohol is a blood thinner). I walked to the mirror so I could wipe my nose.

Apparently at the same time there was a ton of coke on the sink and the attendants assumed it was me because I was wiping off my nose and because they thought I'd just been puking in the stall, so they whisked me to security. They brought me to this big man named Stefan, who accused me of doing coke. I started yelling that I was coughing because of my life-threatening lung disease, that I could die when I'm twenty-five, that I always wear a medical ID bracelet but had taken it off for the party, that doing coke would kill me and I would never EVER do it.

Natasha was there trying to speak to them rationally and soberly, but the guy told her, "You're not helping . . . if you want to help go get her ID because she's going to the police station." She left to get my ID, found Matt and brought him to Stefan, but Stefan ignored him. By this time I was hysterical, crying, telling them that I was protected by the Americans with Disabilities Act and that this was discrimination.

Natasha had the thought to pull out my pills from her bag, which were in a biohazard bag and were clearly prescription pills that looked serious. She said we were guests of Victor and that he would not be happy if he heard about this, and that my dad is a lawyer and HE would not be happy and would try to sue if they took me to the police with no evidence when I was just coughing because of a life-threatening genetic disability.

Finally, he apologized, and then he started sucking up to me and it was insane to see how he changed his act. He was groveling, asking me what I did, said, "You should be a model," and then asked if he could do anything for me. I said no and then started bawling even more. Natasha and Matt helped me calm down. I felt so judged and misunderstood and it just made me realize how what people see on the outside when they look at me is so incredibly different from the reality of who I am.

And I also realized that I should always be wearing a medical ID bracelet, and have a medical card in my wallet to prove to people how serious it is. Always. Because I was so close to ending up at the police and without a sober friend there like Natasha, they would've hauled me to the station. And then I would've had to call my parents from Vegas to explain the situation and that would have been horrific.

The rest of the night was fun, got to bed late, slept like a log, grateful that Natasha was with me.

At the airport they did a full pat-down on me because my machine beeped positive for some bad chemicals or something. Which was just so crazy, second time I felt like a delinquent this weekend. Natasha came to my house for dinner and we told my parents about Vegas.

Today I had an interview with Beth Pratt of National Wildlife Federation, who was so interesting and will be a great resource for the book. Tomorrow I will interview Lili Singer from Theodore Payne Foundation for Wildflowers and Native Plants. Also talking to Garry George from Audubon, Lisa Fimiani from Ballona Wetlands, and Carl Richards (landscape photographer). Also going to look at an apartment in Manhattan Beach with Lauren! It looks like a gorgeous place.

2/17/15
I think I'm more vulnerable than I used to be to the idea of death. I don't know if that's just right now, this very week,

because I'm sick, or if it's just a sensitivity that's increasing over time. Two things spurred this: First, the *Parenthood* finale. The death of Zeek, the grandfather, left me bawling, and not just tears but the entire body shaking kind of bawling. I think it's where my mind wandered that makes me feel unsettled.

When Camille walked in and saw Zeek lying on his chair, and she called to him and he didn't respond, triggered the thought that one day my own parents might have that experience with me, and I thought about how they would feel in that moment and how they would react. It physically pains me to think of it, but I can't not think of it when I see death in any form. And then when they're scattering his ashes, I think about the fact that my own grandpa will die, maybe soon. The emphasis on family is so strong, it makes me realize I don't always express how important my family is to me.

In the show they have flash-forwards to where all the characters are in a few years, new babies, new relationships, family still strong, lives going forward in the most predictable, wonderful way, and I think that that will never be the way my life goes and that makes me sad. Sad for me and for all the people that will be affected. When I get sick, my parents stop their lives. If I were sick to the point that Caleigh is sick, I would feel terrible. It's enough to be scared myself, but to know that my own situation might be taking away happiness from others is devastating.

The second was way more worrisome. I woke up at 6:00 a.m. yesterday and couldn't fall back asleep because I couldn't breathe, had chest pain, and was coughing. I made coffee, did treatment, and then was feeling ambitious (because I was up so early and because of the caffeine), so I drove to CorePower Yoga for a 9:00 a.m. class, which I never get to. It made me happy to be up and out doing something that early. Because of how much time I'm stuck indoors, being out and about in the morning is precious.

I was thinking about how good I have it right now—I'm healthy enough that even when I'm sick, I can move my body and do some exercise. I can get through a hot power yoga class alongside healthy people. I live close to the ocean and can surf. I have incredible friends who I love and have fun with. I have a degree from Stanford. I have incredible family support. I have a new puppy who loves me. The word I've used the most in this paragraph is love—my life is filled with love, with fun experiences, with happiness. And I should have the attitude that I'm so so lucky, and most of the time I do.

But there are moments when it strikes me that all of the things I love will be lost. Breathing will get harder, at some point I'll have to live at home so my parents can help me full-time. A time when I'll get disability money from the government because I can't work. I may or may not find someone who can hang with my disease, who can support me in the way I need to be supported. Sometimes I'm hopeful about that, but oftentimes I'm not, because even if there were people who would be good enough to do it, I might not let them in; even though I seem open about some things, ultimately I'm private, and have never let anyone in. I should not have envy, I recognize that it's a dangerous emotion, but I do for people who have freedom, who can travel, who can see other parts of the world and make their own decisions and do things without worrying that it will drive them to the hospital in the future.

All this thinking led me to the moment where I realized—this might be as good as it gets. It might only get worse from here. When things are going well, I often think something bad is about to come, because I've learned things can only go so well for a limited amount of time. I hate the impending sense of doom, that this goodness I'm living right now cannot last, will not last, that it will be stripped away. The higher you fly, the farther you fall. The healthier I am, the more I start to feel sturdy and strong and capable and normal, the more the slap of reality stings when it knocks me down, shows me my fragility, reminds me that my innards are working against me, not for me.

I thought, if this is as good as it gets, and I died right now, would that be so bad? It's the quit-while-you're-ahead mentality. Obviously I would never act on that. I'm not depressed, I've actually been quite happy and filled with gratitude lately. But I was thinking, if I died right now, it would be like ripping off the Band-Aid. My family and the others who care about me would be devastated. And it would be a huge thing, the thing that happens when people commit suicide where people say, "How could they do this to me? How could they do this to their mother?" etc. I've always been shocked when people say that, because suicide is not about anyone else. It's a last resort for a person who feels they have no other option. That's not how I feel right now.

If I do die soon (from CF) and someone reads this, they might think I was suicidal. But I'm not. I was just thinking about how my death would cause a lot of pain initially, but then my parents and friends could live their lives without having to worry about me, without having to take care of me. It kills me how much pain I might cause others if I die.

Through all of these meandering thoughts, I'm struck by how much more emotionally vulnerable I am than I realized. The fact that I was crying so hard on the way back from yoga that I almost didn't go home (because a song on the radio made me think about suicide) and whether a quick death would save me and my family from pain and suffering. And that my mind went where it did because of a TV show finale makes me realize that my emotional state is fragile.

I'm trying so hard to shift my perspective, to realize that I don't need to be outside of California or far away from family to be happy; I didn't grow up in freaking Minnesota, I grew up in L.A. in a beautiful climate with beautiful nature and beaches nearby, so if I can't climb mountains and surf faraway beaches in Bali and meet indigenous people who are hungry farmers in Brazil, life will still be okay. It's just the fact that those things were taken away from me forcefully by my disease that makes it hard. I might have come to my own conclusion that I'd be happier here in California anyway, but the fact that it wasn't my own choice is the rub.

I need to turn over a new leaf, to start a new, happy life. I'm going to finish Susan's book and do other work that fits my lifestyle. I'm going to meet beachy smart surfer people and have a social life that makes me happy. Maybe I'll meet a guy who is right in every way, who I can finally let myself fall for completely. Maybe I'll live a really long time and decide that having kids isn't a terrible irresponsible choice, and I'll have a family and a dog and a husband, and maybe some medicine will come around that's basically a cure and then CF will just become a maintenance disease instead of a progressive one. Maybe, maybe, maybe.

I need to shut out the impending doom feeling that arrives at the slightest reminder of death. I need to be stronger and not feel like I'm losing my backbone. I'm sick again, and this particular exacerbation has left me terrified, as if this is my first time at the rodeo. It's so normal, it's so routine, but because I wasn't expecting it, it feels harder to process that I might need to go to the hospital again. In Stanford it was routine, expected, almost comfortable (not really, but as close to comfortable as an exacerbation can be).

I was counting on ataluren, living at home, and being in SoCal to escape CF's chokehold. But the hold was still there, just as strong as ever. Letting me have a moment of normalcy, and for that I'm grateful but I'm also pissed. It's playing a game with me and I have to be strong but realistic enough to know that even when I have a period that's good, there's always sickness around the corner and it's not the end of my world. I go in, do IVs, get better. That's what I have to believe for myself, because when I read Caleigh's posts and I think of that as my future, it makes me think that quitting while ahead is easier.

3/17/15

Well, I've emerged from the hellhole of RSV (respiratory syncytial virus, what it turned out I had) and a new chapter is beginning to unfold. I've started moving my stuff into my new Manhattan Beach apartment, which I LOVE. It's two blocks from the beach and I can tell it will be an awesome active lifestyle there. I booked a trip to Hawaii, which is where I am now. This trip is such a trip (like the mind-fuck kind of trip, not a literal trip)—it feels so long since I've been here, but also like no time has passed. The weirdest thing is that the last time I saw Shawn in person we were on such a different level with our friendship, relationship, whatever you want to call it. It's kind of a guessing game as to how to act around him, like whether we're just friends or something more, and I don't know what he wants, whether he still likes me (although I think he still does). I think he's conflicted, I'm conflicted.

Hawaii has been amazing so far. Yesterday, the day we arrived, we gained time so it was a long day but we packed a lot of fun into it!

Today I woke up at 5:00 a.m. naturally—thank you, jet lag! We were in the water from 6:15 to 6:45-ish, and it was stunning.

Incredible. It was dark when we got in the water, the sun hadn't risen yet, so we watched it rise from the canoe in the water. Plus surfing the waves on the canoe was awesome. The water was a gorgeous shade of blue and early-morning surfing has a calmness to it that afternoon surfing does not.

I'm super happy to be here and already feeling so much better in my lungs. Which makes my head feel better. The magical combo of sun and salt makes me recover a lot faster and surfing the warm water in Oahu is the best medicine.

4/7/15

Sometimes I feel like my life is a novel with someone writing it. Making sure there are enough high points and low points, drama and emotion, conflict and resolution. That's why whenever there's a long period of good times, I have the sinking feeling that something bad is to come, that the good, contented stability can't last. Because contented stability doesn't make for a good read.

It also has such distinct chapters, with seemingly abrupt transitions between chapters. One month I'm sick with RSV, living in Beverly Hills, and spending time with my puppy Kona. Then, boom, in Stanford, nervous breakdown about work and life. Then back home, moving stuff to Manhattan Beach apartment, then an unplanned trip to Hawaii.

In Hawaii an abrupt turnaround and I'm feeling better, thrown back into fun with Shawn as if no time had passed, surfing and paddle-boarding, canoeing and volleyball. Then in Maui with Ali and our moms on a mother-daughter getaway, crashing from how much I pushed myself in Oahu, thinking I'll need to be admitted and hoping I can put it off until after a road trip with Shawn. Then back to L.A., living at the beach officially, spending my first night there having so much fun. Then Shawn in town, which was a mind-twister. My two completely separate worlds colliding, then spending time with his family in Santa Ana, going to Club 33 and a day at Disneyland with them and spending the night in his family home.

I need to reflect on how strange and unusual my life is and how book-like it seems and not beat myself up for not journaling more often (even though I want to remember every minute of it).

4/8/15

I just called the clinic to talk to Ronnie* to tell them about my symptoms and my voice was breaking the whole time on the phone. I can't keep it together and it's pathetic. I was sitting outside in the sunshine and feeling sorry for myself, which makes me feel worse because I know it's absurd. And when I hung up the phone after leaving a message, I put my head between my knees and couldn't stop crying. I think these inexplicable tears are more frustrated tears, self-directed, scornful tears, because I think I brought this sickness on myself and now can't deal with it.

My mom saw how stressed I was and mentioned that she could find someone to replace me on Susan's book. The job is an opportunity of a lifetime—to be paid to write about the environment and work for the most awesome woman who is so incredibly understanding about everything in my life and so flexible on deadlines. I can't bear not to finish.

But if I can't even finish one writing job, my first writing job out of college, what hope is there for me to ever not only get another job but have the confidence to look for one? I'm just hemorrhaging my parents' money and my guilt about that makes me sick because they work so hard every day and will work way

---

* the coordinator who took over for Jen when Jen became a nurse practitioner

after they could have retired so that I can have a good life, when I can't even suck it up and work a few hours a day, sick OR healthy.

4/23/15

"We've come to think of healing in mechanical terms, as repairing something broken, like fixing a flat tire. But for most of human history healing has meant more than repairing the body. Healing has meant restoring a sense of wholeness to a person— or even a relationship or community."

This is from the story I produced about cystic fibrosis and the environment, formerly known as "Biome," now called "Salted Wounds." It played yesterday on the podcast State of the Human. The Senior Reflection class and Stanford Storytelling Project are amazing!!

4/29/15

Jesse is writing a song for me!!! She wrote one before, but it was too "happy." CF is a mind-fuck and any song about it should reflect that. I sent her a detailed note about what living with CF is like. Can't wait to see what she does with it!

5/1/15

Spoke today in Margot's Medical Genetics class at Cal State Northridge. It really affected some of the students, hearing my story. They couldn't believe what my life is like. They couldn't reconcile how I look with my reality. Their questions were so widespread; they asked about drug development, my emotional resilience, and what dating with disease was like . . . the whole range.

I was touched that all these people who didn't know me felt like my "speech" made them think I was open enough to answer

those kinds of questions honestly, which I did. It made me want
to do more speaking where I'm not reading from a piece of paper,
but just talking candidly in front of a group of people who actually want to listen and to learn.

I was dreading waking up early for it, driving all the way to
Northridge, etc. But it was totally worth it.

5/26/15

Caleigh is my hero! She was part of a short film for *The Happiness Stories,* a very cool project!

6/8/15

The past few weeks have really started to feel like I live in Manhattan Beach. Like I'm not an impostor when I say I live here. I
have routines. Yoga. Surfing. Volleyball. I've been going to the
grocery store (occasionally) and making food. I've been hanging
out with friends and having so much fun.

7/20/15

Had this idea today that I wanted to write down before it leaves
my mind or I stop feeling inspired or I forget it or something
inside me tells me it's not possible.

I want to start an online media source (podcast? website?) that
tells the stories of people who have struggled with something in
their life and found hope somewhere. Anything from chronic illness to poverty to grief to depression, etc. The hope can be from
anywhere, unexpected places.

Names to consider:

–re: life (about life, but also implying some kind of
renewal/starting over/)
–Project Redemption (or The Redemption Project)

–The hope-knock life (play on words of hope and hard-knock life)

8/29/15

"Breathe deeply, until sweet air extinguishes the burn of fear in your lungs and every breath is a beautiful refusal to become anything less than infinite."

—D. Antoinette Foy

Kari died yesterday. She was a hospital buddy, but more than that, she held a torch that illuminated a new direction for me at a time when my health had left me in a hopeless terror. She was a friend and a fighter with a radiant goodness and fierce compassion, smiling her sweet smile no matter how sick she was. The world became a little bit darker today, when Kari lost her battle with CF. I'm stunned and sickened.

Rest in peace, Kari. So many people loved you. Breathe easy. You are infinite.

9/7/15

I want to get a stick and poke tattoo of the letters LXV—65 in Roman numerals. Caleigh's brother Michael got that tattooed on his inner arm and it looks sick, and I would want to do it on my inner wrist but a lot smaller, so it could be covered with bangles or a watch. I Facebook messaged him to ask how he would feel if I stole his idea and he was like it's totally fine, art isn't owned, I think it would be great if you got it!

10/11/15

Melissa is in the ICU at Stanford, fighting desperately for her life. Now is when it would be good to believe in prayer. She's a mermaid, my soul sister.

10/16/15

I clenched and unclenched, then curled and uncurled my toes as I lay in bed, my torso and neck rigid from my efforts not to cough. With shallow breaths I counted inhales, 1, 2, 3, and exhales, 4, 5, 6, trying to pay attention to the TED Radio Hour podcast I often listen to while falling asleep. On this night, though, at 10:00 p.m. on October 12, 2015, nothing could distract me from my physical pain and discomfort or my emotional anxiety. My throat was sore from the hacking cough I'd had all day, my lungs searing with the pain of pleurisy and infection. My mind was numb from the half-bottle of cough syrup I'd chugged to prevent bronchospasms, but also racing with the fear of what another sleepless night would do to me.

After twenty minutes, I got out of bed and took an Ativan for anxiety. I took a Vicodin for the chest pain, sipped more cough syrup, and did another half-hour breathing treatment. When none of these things provided relief, I knew I could no longer put off going to the emergency room. Physically tense but mentally drugged and fatigued, I called the pulmonary fellow, packed my things, and prepared for another admission. It was a rote going-through-the-motions scenario.

When I was sitting in the waiting room of the ER, waiting to be triaged, the reality of the situation hit me with a staggering force: there I was, the night of my twenty-third birthday, sick, scared, and not even surprised.

Did I ever picture that that is where I would be on my twenty-third birthday? Absolutely not. In life, we often pass the time operating on a scale of minutes and hours. We wait for the bell to ring, signaling the end of a boring lecture. We watch the hours pass at work, waiting for 5:00 p.m. We monitor the timer as we run on the treadmill or the elliptical.

It's rare for us, with our micro-focus on minutes and hours

and days, to zoom out, to step back and ask the big questions: How did I get here? What did I envision for my life, and does my reality match that vision? Or perhaps better questions: How did I not realize, as I got older, that this is where I was destined to be? Why did I let myself envision anything else?

Real change is often made by people who are too young, too inexperienced, or too naive to know that what they're attempting would be considered impossible by others. These folks blindly pioneer and innovate, despite the limitations and restrictions perceived by others. They change the world, even if they fail to do what they set out to do, initially. They change the world by challenging us to look beyond the perceived limitations that we all have, by forcing us out of the boxes we let ourselves get caged in.

In a way, I unwittingly did that for myself. I was sheltered as a child from the brutality of cystic fibrosis, from the likelihood of dying young, from the statistics and stories that say it all. But driven by my own curiosity, I eventually began to seek out stories of patients with *Burkholderia cenocepacia,* the bacteria that colonizes my lungs. They were horror stories—case reports of kids that were healthy one day and dead two weeks later from the rapid necrotizing pneumonia known as cepacia syndrome. I pored over those case reports, then compartmentalized the information, putting it away somewhere in my brain, where I didn't let it affect my decisions or actions.

I managed to remain naive about my future. It never occurred to me that I wouldn't have a career. It never occurred to me that I wouldn't graduate college. It never occurred to me that I wouldn't marry and have a family. It never occurred to me that I could die in my young adulthood. It never occurred to me that when the time came that I needed a lung transplant, I might not be able to get one.

If I had understood the likelihood of any of those things in middle school and high school, would I have dedicated myself to academics and athletics like I did? No. If I had thought I couldn't go to college, I wouldn't have struggled through the difficult concepts in calculus, stressed about AP and honors classes, or done my summer reading. If I had perceived myself as weak and "terminal," I wouldn't have believed I had the strength to play three varsity sports. If I had thought I wasn't going to be around much longer, I wouldn't have formed the lasting friendships that now make up the richest parts of my life. If I hadn't had hope that my future was bright, I would not have stayed resilient throughout months of hospitalizations every year and the inevitable health crises of a chronic illness.

Any time I feel disappointed by my health limitations now, as an adult, I think about the very best parts of my life. In a way, the thing I question most about my upbringing—my naïveté about my illness and the disappointments it inevitably caused down the line—is the quality that made those very best parts of my life possible. It's a trade-off; I've been disappointed at times, but I have also exceeded beyond imagination since I didn't plan for early death.

I wonder sometimes, was it worth it? Should I have been made more aware of my prognosis, been less sheltered from the realities I would face as I aged and my disease progressed? Would that have made things easier or softened the blows as they came?

Most of the time, I think not. The fears I have now that my teenage self didn't have to grapple with allowed me to develop a sense of self before getting slammed with doubts, uncertainties, and anxieties that come with chronic progressive illness. My life may have had fewer surprises, but it would certainly have been less full. And some of the worst surprises in my life have often led to the greatest breakthroughs: extreme disappointments that closed one door simultaneously opened others.

Like many twenty-three-year-olds, I sometimes feel lost and

confused and directionless in my career. Throughout college and in my postgrad life, door after door has been closed to me, career-wise, and more and more things I've desired have become impossible. I just have to hope that one day, after more experience in my freelance writing career, I will feel grateful that those other doors were closed to clear the way for the right one to finally open.

10/19/15

Monday morning, I woke up in my apartment with the pain of a thousand knives collectively stabbing my left mid-back in my left lower lobe. An 8 or 9 on the hospital pain scale—I reserve 10 for being hit by a truck.

My breaths were shallow and quick as I labored to get enough oxygen. After stumbling out of bed, I walked to the coffeemaker, panting and hunching over with my elbow on the counter. *Fuck*, I thought to myself. *I can't do this.* Whether I can get up and make coffee in the morning is a current metric to gauge whether I'm okay or not.

"Mom, I need you to drive down," I said over the phone, sprawled on the bed, searching for a position that would enable me to breathe better. "I'm in pain." I tried not to cry, but my voice cracked.

She came quickly to find me drugged up on Vicodin. My deep breaths and coughs were still excruciating. I've had blood clots in my lungs and the shocking pain of this mundane Monday morning mimicked the pain of those days spent in the ER, discovering infarction and emboli. It occurred to me that I might have another embolism, and that another day in the ER might be in order. A few hours later, I was on my way to the UCLA hospital in Santa Monica, to find out if (medical) history was repeating itself.

Imaging tests done in the ER showed no pulmonary embolism and no collapsed lung. But the pain did have a cause: multifocal pneumonia throughout the lower lobes, with a cavitary lesion on the left side. I had finished a course of IV antibiotics just two weeks prior, and there I was, even worse off than before and ready to begin anew.

When the hospitalist assigned to my case told me I was ready to go home after three days in the hospital, I knew she was wrong. In my gut, I knew that despite my outward appearance of normalcy, my lungs were still embroiled in battle. My body was still crushed with fatigue. And all going home would mean was continuing to undergo the exact same treatment and therapy as in the hospital but being responsible for all of it myself with no help.

Three days in the hospital and two weeks of home IV care later, I returned to my life. But two weeks after that, the crippling pain was back, bringing with it the distinct understanding that someone had fucked up my treatment in a grand way. You don't recover from a pulmonary exacerbation only to develop *pneumonia* (significant, severe pneumonia, according to the doctors) just two weeks later, unless the treatment wasn't right. The fuckup, I think, was a doctor thinking she was doing right by the patient sending her home to recover, when in reality, being sent home before you're ready doesn't fix things. The second fuckup was not listening to me when I said I wasn't ready.

Now I'm back in the hospital again, far worse than I was when I was first admitted. The depth and frequency and force of my cough is frightening, as is the seemingly inexhaustible well of sticky, green, infected mucus I'm producing and expectorating.

Slowly I'm improving, getting weaned off the oxygen supplementation, beginning to get up and walk and stretch my legs, hearing promising reactions from doctors that listen to my lungs, that there's reason to be hopeful.

We can't fully blame a doctor who sends us away, who thinks we're exaggerating our symptoms, even if we end up far sicker than before as a result of treatment cut short. We have to blame the disease, the disease that tries to define us, the disease that none of us asked for, the disease that's killing us, the disease that, no matter how brutal, binds us together.

The year 2015 has been a tough one for the CF community. It's been a month since Kari passed and now it's Melissa who's gone into free fall. Other patients have said it's been an unusually brutal year as they, too, have lost friends to CF.

When someone dies, we all feel the effects, rippling through the network, upsetting the sense of calm that was always an illusion to begin with. We think about them, and how much we'll miss them, and the loved ones that survive them; but we also think about what it means for ourselves, what we can expect, how we can grieve and cope while continuing to care for ourselves.

For months, Melissa and I talked nearly every day. I worried about how sick she was feeling and for how long, but it never once occurred to me that on my twenty-third birthday she would be on life support, and I would be in the emergency room, gasping for breath, begging for relief. It's weird to not be able to talk to her.

She will struggle, but she is mighty and will survive. New lungs will come. And I, with the help of powerful drugs, will beat back the bacteria inflaming and infecting my lungs like one would hack down forest undergrowth with a machete. I have to believe that. For her, for me. For all of us.

10/24/15

Recently, I was running on the treadmill at the gym. More of a slow jog, really, broken up with a minute of walking for every couple of minutes of running. My lungs were searing, and not in a good way. Music was blasting, so I was able to ignore how much my breath was quickening, how erratically my heart was beating. As I slowed to a walk and turned the music down, I felt the spurting feeling I know all too well: like the moment a sprinkler goes off, a blood vessel burst in my lungs and the blood sprayed out, collecting in my airways and gurgling upward to be coughed out.

Staggering off the treadmill, I made my way to the trash can. I hid behind the half-wall, not wanting other gym patrons to think I had tuberculosis (or any kind of contagious illness). I coughed and coughed and spit out fire-engine-red blood into the towels, which I promptly discarded. Then I gathered my water bottle and phone and left the gym, rattled in more ways than one.

Yoga is the antithesis of exercise programs that try to force insecurity on people and make them feel they are not enough. Yoga urges us to take a deep breath, to be grateful for exactly what our bodies can do on a particular day. Yoga reminds us that whatever health we do have is a miracle not to be taken for granted. Yoga restores peace, confidence, and a sense of spaciousness for those who are claustrophobic within the trap of disease. Most of all, it gives us hope.

My first attempt at yoga was a ridiculous haze of movements that felt wrong, positions that felt awkward, stretches that felt painful. I was seventeen then, just out of high school and riding the high of being named by my high school Athlete of the Year all four years of school.

Many women with cystic fibrosis experience a worsening of disease symptoms in their late teens and early twenties. In my case, one or two hospitalizations a year turned into five or six. Friends got used to me popping pills and pushing injections while in the dining room, in lecture halls, and at parties. They got used to me disappearing and did their best to keep me in the loop about life outside of my hospital-home. Acquaintances tended toward confusion at the mismatch between my seemingly healthy outward appearance and the evidence of sickness around me: the needles in my biohazard bin, the catheter in my arm, the syringes sticking out of my purse, the machines filling up my dorm room.

During that horrific period of change and doubt and fear and humility, I was still on a college club volleyball team. The girls were wonderful and the team was competitive. But I couldn't stand that my shrinking lung capacity was shrinking my options, both on and off the court.

So I found my way into a yoga studio. It was Dr. Mohabir's idea to meet me at yoga one night, and for the first time in a long time I experienced the *joy* of movement. I shed my self-loathing, because in yoga, we are on our own journey. With no expectations. We move at our pace. The "coach" guides with gentle suggestions, not commands. Child's pose is always available. And in that particular class, reared back in child's pose while my doctor pumped out chaturangas (planks), I saw myself in the mirror and realized that there is beauty in rest. Endless beauty in not feeling the need to progress. There is a time and a place for progress, but there's a time and a place to yield to the idea of just simply existing.

In the years since my first yoga session, I've had months in which I'm on the mat four times a week and months when I don't practice at all. But it's a safe space, one for which I will always be grateful for showing me self-love, for showing me peace, for showing me the magic in stillness. When I'm too sick to briskly walk a block, I can still get into the studio, as yoga is not about the physical postures; if I enter the room, become present in my physical body, notice the hurts and the sadness and the love and the beauty, if I control my breath in what little way I'm able to, it's a success. Yoga shattered the old parameters and built new ones that I love.

11/3/15

Back in the hospital again. It's the ultimate hamster-on-a-wheel scenario: running to stay in place, never getting ahead, time passing by, giving the perception of motion, but with no ground covered.

11/6/15

It's not the big, groundbreaking health events.

It's not the scariest set of test results.

It's the petty frustrations and humiliations that wear on me, overtax my patience and goodwill, and leave me drained and weakened.

It's that moment when you snap at someone because they're the sixth person to ask you if you're pregnant, even though the urine test already came back negative.

It's when they don't send an RT for seven hours even though you can't breathe and are in distress, but you can't blame anyone in particular because it's "the system."

It's when your IV antibiotic hasn't arrived, because it wasn't ordered. Why not? The dose is weight-based and they don't have your weight, even though they could've taken it at any point during the seven hours you were in the ER.

It's when circumstances are so absurd they defy logic.

It's when the pharmacist tells you that you can't keep certain medications at the bedside, medications you've kept at the bedside every hospitalization.

It's when hospital personnel don't properly gown and glove for your contact isolation status, but then tell your visitors they need to.

It's when you call to ask for hot packs because you're shivering so much it's making you cough up a storm, and twenty minutes later you ask again, and twenty minutes later you ask a third time and they tell you not to use them because you have a fever.

It's when you finally have a minute alone so you break down and cry, and right then someone walks in to take your vitals.

It's when four different people each day ask detailed questions about your bowel movements in front of your visitors.

It's when you feel like you're going to have a panic attack and ask for Ativan, and the doctor on call makes you seem like a drug-seeker and says no.

It's when you want to go to sleep at 9:00 p.m. but can't because the nurse/pharmacy are so late with meds that by the time everything is finally done you can't sleep.

11/20/15
Caleigh is getting new lungs today!!!

11/28/15
As I'm stuck in this hospital, I ponder the ever-nagging question: When to disclose?

In my case, since I grew up in a small bubble in Los Angeles—and went to a K–8 school—my assumption was that everyone knew about my cystic fibrosis early on. They'd heard my cough, seen the high-calorie shakes I chugged in class, watched me pop pills at recess and lunch, noticed I was never in school a full day.

My family was all about disclosure. I never considered that other patients might handle the issue differently. *Mallory's 65 Roses* guaranteed everyone around me knew, since my mom read it to my class each year.

Near the end of high school, I learned of a patient who had such a mild case of CF that she was able to hide it from everyone she knew. She never took pills in front of people, and she hid her airway clearance and nebulizer equipment from friends. I was stunned—when every minute of your day is in some way focused on the physical needs of your body, how can you hide that from the world? Wouldn't that task in and of itself exhaust you until you could no longer keep up the healthy façade?

I took for granted how easy it was when everyone around me already knew about my illness. I liked it that way.

The issue of disclosure became much more pressing for me when I left home, left my tight-knit community for college. On the first day of school, I showed up to my dorm room and began setting up my equipment. Adele and Sabrina, now highly successful medical school students, were intrigued, nonjudgmental, and curious. They had the perfect reaction to rooming with me and it set the tone for me right away that people could hear about my disease and not immediately write me off as either a hyperbolic drama queen or a sickly person that's too diseased to be fun.

Freshman year was a year of introduction frenzy, meeting others in CoHo,* on Wilbur Field, in the dining hall, at a friend's pregame. The people who lived in my dorm saw me do treatment and thus knew about my condition, but people I ate with, partied with, sat in class with, roamed the campus with, didn't ask me

* Stanford Coffee House

about it so I never brought it up. I popped pills all the time, coughed a ton, missed a lot of class (and people talk), so I assumed everyone knew. I found out later on, when I started being hospitalized all the time, that a bunch of people did not know.

Telling people that you have a life-threatening disease has a way of making people extremely uncomfortable. The rare few who respond exactly how I hope they will are usually the ones who become my closest friends. I worry people will view me differently, worry about what they say in front of me, worry what's okay to ask and what things I'd rather not talk about. My preference is for people to ask but I wonder if the burden is on me to disclose.

12/12/15

It's an important day today, the two-month mark from when I got admitted to UCLA hospital for this tumultuous, challenging, soul-testing period. It's been two months since my birthday, which came and went before I had the chance to celebrate. Two months since I've lived within these hospital walls. One year since I was last admitted at Stanford Hospital—a place that felt like home but is now a distant memory. It's amazing how the tricks of time change things, distorting and morphing perceptions and attachments. Now UCLA feels like home.

I fondly remember the days when college friends could visit me at Stanford Hospital. Being in a huge hospital where I could walk thousands of steps, see trees and ducks and water and an extensive collection of beautiful artwork. I could sunbathe and bump into people I knew from school, all without leaving hospital grounds.

But I did leave the grounds during breaks from IVs—sneaking out with my mom daily, walking the ten to fifteen minutes it takes to get to the Stanford Shopping Center. Getting juice from

Pressed, having my hair washed at Hair International, drinking piping hot coconut ginger or masala chai tea from Teavana. Being close enough for my professors (James Campbell, Sue McConnell) to visit. Just being in college—having that sense of purpose, that identity, that attachment to a prestigious university—said enough that people knew I was smart.

I'm tearing from these memories. Not because they're bad, not because they're great, but because they're over. It feels like that period of my life ended abruptly, and not because I wanted it to. I didn't want to let go.

And I figured that when I *did* let go, it would be because I was on my next wild adventure—traveling in New Zealand or Australia, living in Hawaii or San Diego, having a job, literally doing anything besides being in L.A. But the crazy thing is, now that I do live in L.A., I'm entrapped in comfort. Sucked into safety. And not just the emotional safety that drives people to stay close to home: I mean the literal safety of my survival. I don't feel that I'm at a stage of my life where I can afford to live far from my family. They do too much. As much as I hate to admit it, I need them too much. I sacrificed health to go to Stanford—maybe I would have declined no matter what, but I definitely declined more by being away at college. It was worth it, 100 percent worth it. I wouldn't go back and change a thing, except maybe I would delete my period of depression.

When I graduated from Stanford one year ago, I never envisioned that 2015 would pan out the way it did. I fully expected to maintain my connection to Stanford, both through close college friendships and by frequent visits to see doctors once every month or so. I figured whenever I needed to be admitted, it would be there. I did not realize that I would live in L.A., and that when I got sick, I would need to be hospitalized here—that flying back would be too dangerous. I figured my care in L.A. was temporary and I would either stick with Stanford or switch to San Diego (if I decide to move there).

But now, more than ever before, my life is dominated by fear. No, that's too extreme. I don't feel fear in every moment. It's my decisions that are driven by fear. My decision not to get a part-time job and just freelance is driven by fear. My decision not to move to San Diego is driven by my fear of living in a new city alone, too far from my family and Kona.

I'm listening to Trevor Hall's new album right now in my hospital room, alone at UCLA (which is rare, and right now, appreciated), mourning this transition. I'm happy here (as happy as one can be spending two months in a hospital) so it's not that I'm suffering, nor do I think Stanford is the only place for me. It was just my place. My home. And when you lose a home you have to mourn it, which is something I haven't had the chance to do—mostly because before this period, the transition didn't feel complete. Now, with the entire staff of Izzy's Deli knowing me from my daily visits, and the hospital staff recognizing me from taking care of me for so long, this is my new place, and I know that it's a good place.

Being in the hospital this much does weird things to your brain. It's almost scary that it feels so normal to be here, that being out of the hospital is what feels unnatural. The idea of being at my apartment, for example. The last time I was there for any period longer than a couple of days, Micah was there! He was supposed to be there temporarily but decided to stay. I've been there when my new roommates lived there, but that doesn't feel like the norm yet. And taking care of myself, doing everything on my own plus going back to working—that feels incredibly intimidating after being taken care of in the hospital for so long. It's a big day in here if I get to take a shower and do an hour of "exercise"—how am I going to tack on all the time needed to do my treatments, take care of all my meds/sinus rinses, clean equipment, and deal with pharmacies? PLUS work, PLUS exercise, PLUS trying to have a social life? It's too much. And if that feels like too much, how the hell am I ever going to add anything into my life?

I'm going a little bit crazy in here. I need to just get out and into my life and stop thinking about it.

12/15/15

I never thought I would say this, but I've come to love the feeling of being on opioids. It was never part of my treatment but as my chest pain became unbearable I needed it to breathe. With morphine and oxy there's no pain and no sadness. I don't take pain meds when I don't need them, but my pain came back last night for a little bit, and it was not that severe but verging, so I took the smallest dose of oxy. I'm scared of myself a little bit. A lot of the time I feel normal, but then sometimes when I think about things, I'm like, "I want to get some oxy to have on hand just in case I have pain," which I think is valid, but then I wonder if it were just sitting in my drawer, and if I were having a bad day . . . I don't want to put myself in any situation for possible abuse. And I never thought I was at risk before. But now I realize it can really happen to anyone and I need to be careful, and I'm happy the doctors don't want to send me home with oxy. They say if I have pain that severe, I should come to the ER. It's a valid point.

12/16/15

Oh Happy Days, I'm getting out—we're heading home!!!

12/19/15

I've started working again this week and it's nice, it's bringing my brain back from the dead. The first day was so hard . . .

looking at my notes made me anxious, because I forgot where I was and couldn't figure out what next step to take. It felt overwhelming. All my information and research were scattered. I wished the interviews I did with Scott Logan and Garrison Frost were already transcribed and started beating myself up for not having transcribed them, and then beating myself up for not having done enough research, not talking to the right people, not knowing enough about plants. But slowly I just got into it, sentence by sentence, and tried to maintain patience. I reminded myself of the central message of *Bird by Bird* (by Anne Lamott). James Clear sums it up simply: "To become a better writer, you have to write more. Writing reveals the story because you have to write to figure out what you're writing about. Don't judge your initial work too harshly because every writer has terrible first drafts."

Now, it's my third day working, and I have a good flow going. I don't know that I'll finish by the self-imposed deadline of Dec. 30, but as long as I am working every single day toward that goal, I feel okay about it.

Today I had a really nice time with the Sadwick sisters and my cousin Clara. Rebecca and Ari brought their sister Kayla. We went to Fonuts for hours. It was nice to be out of the house. It was a beautiful day; we had pastries and coffee.

The whole time I was getting calls from Coram Home Health* because I need a PICC line dressing change and they haven't been responsive. I called them twice yesterday, Friday, because that was the day I needed it and they promised a nurse would get in touch with me. No nurse called. I called back this morning and told my contact that it was urgent, and I needed the dressing changed today. He said he would call a nurse. A nurse did

---

* Coram has since been acquired by CVS Pharmacy.

call, but she said she didn't have any supplies and that I would need to get supplies from Coram. I had her call Coram to ask. Coram called me back and asked what I needed, and I explained everything. Then another nurse called and we went through it all again. Coram called back yet again to get the exact specifics of what I did and didn't need. I asked when the supplies would arrive and they said they couldn't give an exact time (of course; they claim that every single time) but that it would be sometime tonight. I thought everything was settled. I figured the worst thing that might happen would be that I'd have to stay in tonight, waiting for supplies and the nurse.

Then at 1:45, Daniel from Coram calls back and says, we can't get this for you because you're no longer on our service. You switched to a different pharmacy so it's their responsibility; we are not involved and can't help you. I said that the other pharmacy was not an infusion pharmacy and would not have these supplies *and* that they're closed on weekends so I wouldn't be able to get anything from them for days. He said he would call his manager.

He finally called back and said the manager said no. I asked him if he heard me when I said my local pharmacy was closed on the weekends. He said, well, they agreed to take over, so they need to do this for you. I said, that's inconsistent because Coram agreed to send me two weeks' worth of tubing even *after* I had switched to the local pharmacy, so it was within the manager's power to say yes. He continued to say no. I said, what you're telling me is that you don't give a shit, you'd rather I get an infection and have it go into my blood and threaten my life than get me these goddamn supplies. He said, it's your local pharmacy's responsibility. I repeated myself, said they are closed and it's your fuckup that drove me to them in the first place. He said, there's nothing we can do, this is my manager's final decision. I told him to connect me to the manager. He said, there's no way to contact her except on her personal cell, so I said, give me that then. I said, someone above the person answering the phone is available today and you need to connect me. He said no. I asked him to give me his full name and the full name of his manager and said my dad would call them and that I was a LOT nicer than my dad would be. He put me on hold for ten minutes before I finally hung up. I was shaking.

During this conversation I asked him if he was aware that he worked for a *healthcare* company. I told him his company was responsible for jeopardizing my health due to false promises and failure to follow through on them. It's outrageous that they didn't tell me thirty hours prior, the first time I called about my dressing change, that they couldn't help me.

I started out nice. I could have started by being accusatory and demanding but I wasn't. I told him his company had screwed up badly and driven me to another pharmacy, but that I was not going to take my anger out on him. But then he turned out to be just another one of those assholes. I finally paged the doctor at UCLA so that the on-call hospitalist could write new orders to Coram or another infusion pharmacy to get me supplies today. But right after I spoke to the doctor, the first nurse from the morning called back and told me she had the supplies. I was relieved, but also pissed because she could have told me that five hours earlier and saved me so much stress, anger, and time wasted on the phone, yelling at an idiot who was never going to be convinced that my life was more important than his manager's indifference and laziness.

I wish I could testify against them in court. I wish I could explain in detail every single mistake they've made and every single way they've made my life ten times more complicated than it needs to be. I wish I could just check back into the hospital (not really, but right now I do) because then I wouldn't have to fight every minute of every day for what I need. It's devastating, criminal in fact. And a reminder that they shouldn't discharge patients from the hospital until home healthcare is worked out perfectly. Staying in the hospital another day would be a small price to pay to avoid this deep distress.

12/25/15

No progress so far on the New Year's resolutions, or even productive reflections about this year and what went well, what went wrong. Going to try an internal dialogue, but I'm setting my expectations very low.

Why do I write New Year's resolutions?

Because I want to stop feeling aimless. I want to take control over my life and actually determine where I'm going. I want to feel consistently happy again. I need to search the deepest trenches of my soul to figure out how to get there. Maybe going back to the concept of a North Star would be more useful than New Year's resolutions since resolutions seem to emphasize achievements rather than habits and processes. Like the destination, rather than the journey . . . ?

Gonna try that. My North Stars are:

Happiness
Meaning
Productive work
Strong relationships that nourish, not deplete
Community
Routines that ground and energize me
Self-assuredness, mental health
Health (Maybe this shouldn't be a North Star, since it's not my choice whether I'm healthy or sick? Have to think about this one.)

Treatment compliance
Exercise
Nutrition
Sleep
Youth, Spontaneity, and Adventure (lacking in this depart-
ment, must balance this with health)
Friends
Family

A better metaphor for this than North Star might be *pillars*.
Pillars that would make my life good.

2016

1/2/16

I had a great New Year's Eve and a great New Year's Day. I went
to a pregame party with a bunch of people I haven't seen in a
long time, then to the Snapchat party downtown. It was like a
big Stanford reunion crossed with a ritzy bar mitzvah, and Fos-
ter the People played. It was nice to feel like a normal person.
But it also reminded me how much of my life and myself I've
lost recently, because people would ask me how I've been, what
I've been up to, and I either had to lie or just be really vague so
I wouldn't be a downer. One guy mentioned that he's seen on
Facebook that I've been in and out of the hospital a lot and I was
so awkward in my response. I was just like, "Yeah, it's been
tough but it will be okay."

But it was great to hang out, doing what I should be doing

at twenty-three. At the actual party I realized how much of a grandma I am (not that I didn't already know). It was nice to mingle but after a certain amount of time, the venue was too loud and too crowded, and I felt claustrophobic. I was tired and I wanted to go home. I left at 11:50. It was a great night, though.

Unfortunately, I didn't fall asleep until 4:00 a.m., so I couldn't get up at 8:00 a.m. the next morning to be ready to drive to the Rose Bowl with friends. I went later with my parents, and Linda and Steve. When we got there, we went to the alumni tailgate, so we saw a bunch of people, ate food, etc. It was fun and warm. Best part of the day!

Stanford demolished Iowa so it wasn't the most exciting game but I don't get football anyway. I was just extremely happy to be there and so grateful to be out of the hospital. It was a beautiful day and I can understand now why some people choose to live in Pasadena. Middle of winter and it was a gorgeous, clear day, and so green, with mountains on all sides.

We left with four minutes on the clock. I was exhausted and slept twelve hours that night.

The next day was not good. I started coughing up blood and it was a much bigger bleed than usual (30 ccs), causing me to vomit a bunch of times. I was sitting in the bathroom on the edge of the tub, alternating between coughing blood into a cup and then vomiting into the toilet. It was quite a sight. At that moment, I was filled with an overwhelming sense of hopelessness.

When I coughed another 20 to 25 ccs of blood that night, we knew to go to the ER.

All things considered, it was a smooth ER trip that ended with an admission. But I was an emotional mess. I gave Kona a big hug before I left but wished he could come with me.

1/5/16

Still in the hospital. My head hurts and my body is heavy with stress. At midnight I coughed up 10 ccs of blood, then 50 ccs, 70 ccs. They moved me to the ICU and ordered a CT scan.

1/9/16

Life in the ICU is a whole different world. The toilet in the middle of the room with no walls around it strips me of my dignity and, combined with my multiple meds that cause constipation, it's impossible to have a bowel movement. When I first got moved back to intermediate ICU on Thursday afternoon, I was ready to kiss the ground of my familiar room 5498. I was relieved, and it felt like the first moment in days that I could take a deep, non-agitated breath.

I can't believe Melissa spent eighty days in the ICU at Stanford. How did she suffer through that for so long? Two days or so in there changed me. Michelle commented that she could tell I was pissed at one of the nurses. I was surprised. I said, I'm not pissed at her, what made you think that? And she said, you're normally so sweet to the nurses but this time I could see your irritation on your face.

It's not the nurses' fault—in fact, they're super attentive, and the ones I had were very sweet. But the ICU policies make me insane when I feel like they are hindering my health instead of helping it.

I was psyched to get back to 5498. Natalie and Liana came to visit. When I didn't have the energy to hang out anymore, I rolled over to take a nap. When I awakened I stood up to pee and wash my face. I stretched my arms overhead and it raised my heart rate a tiny bit . . . then I felt the familiar gurgling sound, and my heart just sank.

I only coughed up 10 ccs of blood but it was enough for my mom and the docs to freak out. I had been about to take a shower —they were going to change my port needle, so I'd had them pull out my extra IV, and I was more excited for that shower than I think I have been for anything in the last few months. It had been so long, I was caked in grime. I was smelly and hairy and dread-locked. I needed the catharsis of the hot water and solitude. And I had been waiting patiently but desperately for forty-eight hours for that shower: it had been planned down to the minute, since with four IV drugs that each run for one to four hours, there hadn't been a minute when I wasn't hooked up to some IV. This was my only chance. I had a half-hour window locked and loaded but I coughed up blood right at the beginning of that window.

The doctor rounding said no shower. I started crying when he said that and so my mom nicely asked the doctor to think about the whole patient. She told him I was losing my mojo, that this shower meant more to me than he could imagine. He said he would send a colleague to check me out.

His colleague, Dr. Bierer, the ICU intensivist for the night, came by. We talked for a while. He said showering probably wasn't a good idea because of the humidity. I said I didn't have a problem with humidity and told him that I would sit down in the shower on a bench and that the care partner could be in there to watch me. I said, all my vitals are stable. He finally caved and said okay.

In the shower, I scrubbed off the grime and dead skin and anger. The washcloths were brown after scrubbing one limb! I sat on the bench and while I didn't have the total privacy and solitude I craved, I had the hot-water catharsis I needed. It's a reliable, dependable sort of healing. When I came out, I was rejuvenated and way less distraught.

They said if I had any more bleeding that night, they would move me back to the ICU. They said they thought it would be best to move forward with embolization. I fell asleep last night on NPO* assuming I would start hearing about the timing for embolization in the morning.

But when Friday morning came, I couldn't drink my coffee, and no one came by. A couple of hours later I fell back asleep for three hours, and during those hours, I know my mom was harassing the nurse and the doctors, trying to get Interventional Radiology to come up and do a consult to figure out the procedure time. After getting nowhere, the resident under Dr. Paull told my mom that I could eat because it was Friday afternoon and the procedure probably wouldn't happen. He said they wouldn't want to do it so close to the weekend. My mom was rightly pissed. She asked my nurse to page Dr. Paull just as the IR team came for a consult, so I woke up.

Dr. Lee, the IR head guy, started talking about all the risks of the embolization procedure and how I don't meet the standard guideline of 240 ccs hemoptysis all at once. He said, based on the risks and the fact that I wasn't having life-threatening, emergent hemoptysis at that time, he didn't recommend the procedure. Eshaghian was my main doctor and as the head of CF she knew more about this than anyone else.

I made Dr. Eshaghian's case for her: I've had over 240 ccs hemoptysis cumulative over the course of a few days and so have had to stop all treatments. The chronic, lifelong infection will never go away; we've been aggressively treating my infections with antibiotics, but they're not really working, and I've been in and out of the hospital for months. And the longer I go without treatments, the worse the infection gets, and then the worse the bleeding gets. He heard me out, then Dr. Paull came in and explained to Dr. Lee that my doctors were recommending the pro-

* no food or fluids by mouth

cedure, and then Dr. Eshaghian got on the phone with Dr. Lee and explained her thought process and why she really thought I should get it done.

Finally, they said, okay, we're doing it. A few hours later, I got wheeled down to the O.R. I was nervous but also excited to get it over with. Dr. Lee was very nice and said he was going to take very good care of me. A nurse named Jason told me he was going to be responsible for my anesthesia, monitoring my vitals, etc. He told me I wouldn't be fully asleep because they'd need to communicate with me during the procedure, but that he would make me comfortable.

At one point they had to pull my pants off and expose my whole lower half, naked on the table, and one of them apologized that the room was all men. The reason for removing my pants was to go through an artery in the groin to get to the lungs. At that point I felt very scared and stressed out. I was in a cold room on a skinny table (a table that felt too skinny even for me). I was alone in a room full of men, with my vagina completely exposed. People were coming in and out and getting ready, and I was just naked, getting my groin area cleaned with betadine. I was struck by the absurdity of it. Thankfully Jason came and gave me IV Benadryl first, then they got me sort of covered up with a sterile tent thing, and then they gave me either fentanyl or Versed, I don't know which one.

The whole thing took over three hours. By the end I was fully awake and had to go through the nudity thing again. The IR fellow had to close up the incision with this collagen injection thing that was pretty uncomfortable, then he had to hold pressure on it for a long time, and all while I was exposed. He talked to me throughout the time that he was applying pressure, which distracted me, and he explained what he was doing as he closed the incision.

Eventually Dr. Lee came back and checked my ability to move, making sure I wasn't paralyzed. He told me the procedure went well. He said that although he had been hesitant in the morning, after going in there, he was sure that it had been the right thing to do. He embolized five blood vessels, I think, more than he thought he would have to. The only complication was that a piece of wire broke off. He said it shouldn't cause any problems because it's in vessels that are now dead anyway, but he had to keep me informed and he was going to write to the company about it because pieces of wire should not be breaking off inside the body.

Then they put a dressing on my wound, got me clothed, and I said goodbye to them all. They were a good team and I would give them five stars if one reviewed surgical teams on Yelp.

Overall, I'm extremely relieved the procedure is over. Pain is a small price to pay for the certainty of knowing I won't bleed from that spot anymore or have to go back to the ICU, for now, anyway.

1/12/16

In some ways what's going on feels like déjà vu. It reminds me of my senior year of high school. The parallels are that I'm at UCLA, my docs think I might have cepacia syndrome, I've been on IVs for a long time, I keep losing weight, and we're talking about transplant.

Beyond these similarities, this feels like uncharted territory. For one thing, I now judge people for the things they say when they're just trying to be nice (don't worry, it will get better! or other similarly clueless comments). I explode at my mom for little things and am always on the verge of tears. I'm glued to Netflix for mindless time-passing; Facebook; Instagram. Yet I can't bring myself to do anything actually productive (like journaling more, or writing something publishable, or doing actual work that I could get paid for).

The truth is I'm scared. Not in the active acute way you'd be if a rapist were chasing you, but in a chronic, subconscious way that eats at my identity. If I went back and read my journals from sophomore and junior years at Stanford, I'd probably see identical language—about loss of identity, loss of purpose, fear, depression. But thinking back to that point, I was living on campus, going to classes, getting good grades, and I was constantly surrounded by people, so even though I felt extremely lonely and scared, I was moving forward in life. Now my life is completely stagnant. I'm losing time. Not moving forward toward anything. Not getting stronger from all the things that supposedly "don't kill you but make you stronger." I feel like each individual blow is weakening me, and collectively they are causing the foundation of my being to crumble.

None of this reflection feels fresh, it's the recycled dregs, the churned-up feelings that I'm now realizing are familiar. They're the feelings I have and the words I use whenever I'm going through a period that threatens the idea of my future. When I feel the weight of my mortality crushing me, making me wonder if there's anything left in me besides the identity of "sick girl."

In micro moments I can be okay. I woke up this morning feeling fairly optimistic—my pain was not horrible, and my O_2 was good. I drank my coffee, read my book. Then I coughed up 10 ccs of blood—which scared me. Another day of withholding treatments.

When Dr. Eshaghian came, we talked for a long time about whether to resume ataluren or not, about the bleeding, about my need for a blood transfusion.

For a few days she had asked me to hold the ataluren since she wasn't sure if it was associated with the bleeding. But then when

I kept bleeding after being off it a few days, she said she was okay with me going back on it.

The ataluren question still weighs on me. On the one hand, I don't want to ignore Dr. Mohabir's advice. I think his word is the word of God: when he told me not to move to Hawaii, which I had my heart set on, I changed my entire postgrad plan. I trust him with my life. If I were dying, I'd want him on the case. And he's telling me that he wants to abolish ataluren from my medical regimen. His argument is that there's not enough evidence to rule out ataluren being the cause of my hemoptysis or increased complications. The problem is I've tried it twice and both times was so much better. Dr. E is open to continue using it since I seem to do better on it.

1/29/16

Tomorrow marks four weeks within hospital walls with just a few days out. This unexpected and lengthy hospitalization knocked the wind out of me (double meaning intended). In the first three days of the new year, I spent hours reflecting on the previous months of sickness and anchoring myself in the belief that 2016 would be "better."

Since 2015 took the reins away from me, I was determined to get them back. I wanted to go back to living in my apartment in the South Bay, working as a freelance writer, surfing and playing volleyball in my spare time, and fighting every day for continued health. My understanding of the impermanence of circumstances was the beacon that got me through 2015.

But CF is not impermanent. This or that particular hospitalization was—the one where I could work out in the courtyard, the one where I was bedridden; the one where I had many visitors, the one where I refused company; the one where I laughed and ate and walked and did headstands, and the one where my pain and breathlessness stole my vitality. But since I'm not an idiot, and since humans have the ability to make reasonable pre- dictions about the future based on past experiences, I know that variations of these situations will always be a part of my life. And that's the hardest fact I have to grapple with in scary times.

My fight for control over CF is a struggle I will always bear, no matter how much my experiences tell me it's a fruitless one. Each year when most people tell themselves they're going to join a gym or eat healthier or lose weight, I tell myself that I'm going to have a less tumultuous year coexisting with my illness.

2/3/16

During my lengthy hospitalization, the dark voices in my head, brokers of hopelessness, were countered by conversations with Danielle. Never a dealer in unwarranted optimism, she validated my fears and offered some much-needed perspective. We dis- cussed advanced care planning and my end-of-life preferences, as I watched CF friends reach the cusp of death while facing life-threatening complications myself. Danielle told me about Voicing My Choices, a tool for patients to express what would be important to them at the end, should they not be able to communicate themselves. I learned how to effectively manage pain from her and how to advocate for my own palliative care needs with the doctors at my hospital. We talked about grief and fear and coming to terms with a prognosis that's dire and scary. She slept on a chair in my ICU room many nights, driving after work from one hospital to stay with me in another.

The details of many of our most significant conversations during the darkest time are lost in an opioid-induced haze, but the emotional impact of having a friend who does palliative care social work will always stay with me. Danielle is able to apprehend my concerns, and challenges me to conceptualize my circumstances in new ways. One night, as we talked about death and the impact of dying on family members, she gave me an apt metaphor for a coping mechanism: compartmentalizing grief and fear into a box, with a lid, and then opening and closing that box. It's healthy to open the box sometimes and explore and sit with those feelings, but then to be able to close it so that the darkness doesn't cast a shadow over the time one does have left.

She was able to listen and offer wisdom in a way that normal friends cannot; hard as they may try, most will never understand what it means to live with an invisible fatal illness. The balance of validation and perspective that comes from someone who's seen hundreds of families going through similar struggles helped me simultaneously accept the probability of more pain in the future and feel more grateful about what health and time I have left.

2/4/16

This January will be remembered as the month of ten-ish bouts of serious hemoptysis, worsening and severe anemia, one blood transfusion, three rounds of IVIg (immunoglobulin therapy), two doses of FFP,* two bronchial artery embolizations, a large hematoma (a complication of the embolization that left me bed-ridden), severe pleuritic lung pain, around-the-clock opiates and nausea medication, vomiting, an inability to eat for two weeks, two bronchoscopies, two CT scans, many X-rays, discussion of transplant, two stints in the ICU, five hospital rooms, and over a dozen caring and brilliant doctors on my case.

It's been eventful!

Throughout this medical saga, I have relied on so many capable doctors and nurses and care partners to get me through. Ashley, the nurse who washed my hair in the ICU when I couldn't

---

* fresh frozen plasma

get out of bed, went so above and beyond the call of duty, she should get a gold star and a raise. In this hospital I've called home for so many months, I see housekeepers and transporters and EKG techs and care partners and nurses and cafeteria workers/ cashiers and families of other patients and attendings/fellows/ residents that all cheer me on as I walk in my halting and slow way around the floors and courtyards. I saw a family member of another ICU patient in the elevator and she flashed a huge smile and gave an air high five at the sight of me walking, sans heart monitor, oxygen tank, walker, and emergency wheelchair.

With my discharge planned for this coming Monday, I think about rejoining life beyond the hospital's walls and am struck by that most banal of observations: no matter who we are, our time is limited. There's no time not to enjoy every single day, because the days go by so damn fast. One-twelfth of this new year has passed, and I have eleven-twelfths left to take control over my life's narrative.

We are the writers of our own story. That our story will someday end is inevitable for all of us, but the way we get there is not. The piece that's often lost on us, though, is that our level of control extends to how we react to situations, not necessarily to the situations that arise. My effort to thread that awareness into my narrative begins with this understanding and will continue with each and every moment I decide to love the present instead of pining for lost opportunities.

Instead of trying to enforce health as a New Year's resolution, I will try to enforce an unwavering embrace of the messy, impermanent, underrated present. I'm ready to rejoin my other life, but this hospital life is not the worst.

2/10/16
One of the things I worry about now is opiate dependence and

the fact that pleuritic chest pain will probably be a part of my life in all my future exacerbations. Growing up, severe pain was not a problem for me. The first time I started having serious chest pain was when I had pulmonary emboli . . . so for a while after that, I was always worried about either an embolism or a pneumothorax (collapsed lung) when I got severe chest pain. But now, for the last six months, I've had chest pain as a regular part of my symptom list, usually correlating with pneumonia.

The pain that comes is so severe, I can't do anything—can't think/breathe/move/sleep because there's no way to ignore it. It makes me curl up into a hunchback, trying to take shallow breaths so that I won't feel the pain. It's horrible. And it can last for days, a week, two weeks. This past hospitalization, when I had two weeks of severe pain from the hematoma, followed by another week of severe pleuritic lung pain, I was on high doses of opiates for three weeks. We tried a bunch of different combinations, including the opiates morphine, Dilaudid (hydromorphone hydrochloride), Norco (Vicodin), Oxycontin, Percocet, etc., and then other non-opiates like increased gabapentin (for nerve pain), lidocaine patches, and a muscle relaxant.

The pain management team consisted of a really sweet attending and a terrible fellow. The fellow seemed skeptical of my motives and my pain. He kept telling me that it was going to be really hard to get off the drugs and said he didn't want to increase my dose when my pain was bearable because it would threaten my eligibility for transplant. Which is an INSANE thing to say to someone who is in severe pain and who isn't even ON a list for a transplant anywhere—someone who may not be eligible for transplant at any point in the future because of resistant bacteria or too low of a BMI (body mass index).

· · ·

I still can't really process what happened. The constant upheaval of getting admitted, then adapting to hospital life, then getting released is giving me whiplash. My life feels like a disorganized shit show. I think I need a motivational life coach to help me get my affairs in order: to help me get organized, help me finish the book project, help me toward my goal of financial independence, etc. Those are lofty goals, though. For right now, I just need to stay out of the hospital for longer than a week.

But happily I'm writing this from home, having had a super fun weekend. Natasha is in town. We went to the beach Saturday and later played games with the usual suspects (chill night), and Sunday spent all day at the beach again. Being back at my apartment felt so familiar and so foreign at the same time. Weird. It will take getting used to, for sure, but I'm so excited to be back there.

2/20/16

It's been eighteen days that I've been out of the hospital. Eighteen days!! That's the longest time I've spent out of the hospital since October. Granted I'm still on round-the-clock home IVs, but I'm out living in the world.

And I'm moving to San Francisco. I went to Stanford on the ninth and saw Dr. Mohabir on the tenth, and he worked hard to convince me that I needed to be under his care again. Some of what we discussed:

> Hemoptysis—he says it's deadly, seen too many patients die from it, wants to make getting control of it a priority
> Ataluren—his insistence I go off it
> My thinking—he says not to focus on long-term lung function but instead, the possibility that I have cepacia syndrome and how to treat

Scheduling—he wants me in clinic every one to two
weeks for six months to get me stable and back on
track
L.A.—he says flying/driving up to see him every two
weeks not workable; that I need to move back up
Marinol—he's open to starting medical marijuana pills to
decrease nausea/pain and increase appetite
Nausea/vomiting—need to get that in check
UCLA regimen—will continue for now minus ataluren

He said he would respect whatever decision I made in terms
of where to live but made it clear that he's the one with the most
expertise to treat me. UCLA has no other patients with *cepacia*.
I'm the only one. He's impressed with Dr. Eshaghian and said the
infectious disease docs are great, but they just haven't seen enough
cepacia cases.

I was holding it together until the parking lot. My dad gave
me a hug and said he would stand by my decision. I started bawling and said that I couldn't make the decision myself, I didn't
know what to do. I knew that I would agonize over the decision.
Moving again seemed so stressful. He said, "Okay, I'll decide for
you, you're moving."

The day was really significant because my dad had been the
most upset about Mohabir's dislike of ataluren and thought his
position was wrong. It was good that he came to the appointment
because he got to hear the argument from the doctor himself instead of hearing it indirectly through my mom. He became convinced that I should go off ataluren and move up there. We called
my mom and told her. She didn't seem surprised and I came to
find out she and Dr. Mohabir had discussed it all before. She had
had my dad go with me (very unusual) since he's the one that

understands the medicine and she wanted to make sure he agreed with the plan. She canceled her dinner plans and started looking and found me an apartment online while I was still grieving the fact I had to leave Manhattan Beach. She asked my dad to see it the next day. Within twenty-four hours I had an apartment to move to. I went online to find a roommate. Ari responded immediately!

Since then I've adjusted to the idea but am stressed about moving. Very sad to leave the beach but my vision of going back to life the way it was last summer, before I got sick, was not worth clinging to with my health so compromised.

I'm severely atrophied. Starting to gain weight and hoping to turn some of that into muscle. It's hard to build muscle if you have no excess fat, so people have told me not to start working out until I gain some fat. It's unreal, though—I went to yoga the other day, to a class that would've been so easy eight months ago and kept up for about 5 percent of the class but spent the other 95 percent on my back, in forward fold, or in child's pose. The instructor even came over to ask if I was okay, and I said, I'm okay; I just spent a long stretch in the hospital so I'm taking it easy and I'm here for the stretching. She looked shocked and just told me to do whatever felt right. That's precisely why I like yoga. If it was another type of class, the instructor would have said I shouldn't be there.

I am excited for some independence. But also terrified. I know I'll miss my family and be homesick at first, especially for Kona! Will miss my mom popping over with food and hanging out for an hour, taking me to Costco, etc. But it will be good for me to be on my own because I know I rely on my mom and dad way too much.

Will start making a photo book to thank them for all their help.

3/6/16

I moved! It's been such a whirlwind. The surprise was that leaving my apartment was less emotional than I thought it would be. It's as if my heart was already out the door and all we had left to do was remove my stuff.

3/11/16

It's been almost two weeks that I've been in S.F. and it's amazing so far. I love waking up in my apartment, opening the blinds, seeing the trees, the water, and the Golden Gate Bridge, the morning light filling the room. Then making my coffee and sitting in the kitchen or living room. Drinking my coffee and eating breakfast. Small rituals that mean so much. In just two weeks I already feel like I have more of a routine than I did in Manhattan Beach.

I've been going to the gym every day; don't remember the last time I skipped a day. It's so nice there, I can create good workouts for myself, and I'm definitely getting stronger. Curious to see what my lung function is next week. I think my weight is going up, probably as a result of working out and gaining muscle mass. At the gym yesterday I weighed 145 and supposedly had 11.2 percent body fat. My period is still not regular, though, so it might be low.

I was sad when my parents left. It was nice having them here and they did SO much for me. This whole move was only possible because of their involvement. But now it's time for me to accomplish things—starting with making a daily schedule, writing a to-do list, getting it done, going to the market, cooking for myself, cleaning for myself, scheduling my medical appointments and my drug refills/deliveries, etc. All the little things of daily life that my parents helped me do before. It made me feel incompetent, but at the same time I needed their help.

3/24/16

Going on four weeks in S.F. now. It feels like I got to hit the reset button after the worst health period of my life. Yesterday marked seven weeks out of the hospital and I have trouble comprehending how lucky I am, after more than six months of never staying out longer than a week or two. I'm getting used to the idea of waking up each morning not wondering if I'll have to go to the ER that day.

This move puts a healthy distance between the worst health period of my life and my newfound semi-stability. But I'm worried about Caleigh. She's in the hospital post-transplant with a crazy infection in her left lung that showed up as a huge mass on her CT scan. Hearing how hard things are for her right now reminds me how lucky I am. And how unpredictable this disease is.

This apartment, this city, and this lifestyle are so much better for me right now, when I'm on IVs. I'm surrounded by friends so I'm never lonely—except that I ache for Kona whenever I see a dog, and I miss my parents and Maria. I FaceTimed my mom the other day so I could see Kona, but when he heard my voice, he started freaking out and looking for me. I worry that he's never actually going to come up here and that he's going to forget about me and he's not going to be MY dog anymore. Also, times like today, when I'm sick and hanging out at home, I really wish he were here.

Still going to the gym frequently! I've been trying different classes. Mostly yoga, but I did a class the other day called Best Butt Ever, haha. And Barre yesterday, which I liked a lot because it reminded me of Pilates. It didn't make me sweat but still made my muscles burn and incorporated a lot of stretching.

I went to a concert on Tuesday and had a lot of fun, so I'm going to another concert on Sunday. And then two Tuesdays from now, I'm going to a concert at Jason's apartment!

4/2/16

Read a book with a character that resonates with me. Ina describes that when she became an adult, she felt like a failure because she struggled so much with balancing the responsibilities of work, life, etc., and her mother had made it all look too easy, like a superwoman. In a similar way, my mom sleeps five to six hours a night, wakes up energetic, conquers the gym by 8:00 a.m., works all day, juggles hundreds of friends, manages a household, was a hands-on mom, takes care of her parents, and is a master problem-solver. She just gets shit done and has remarkable energy and that's just not my personality. I don't have a lot of energy, I need way more sleep, I can't just go-go-go. It all just feels inadequate when I look at what other people can do, but especially my mom.

Her role was to be in charge all the time. She set it up that way and wouldn't have had it any other way

She worked inside and outside the home, more often at home as I got older, but she always had meetings out of the house. It made it seem to me that working was the normal thing to do, BUT that being there for your kid whenever they might need you was also normal. It was this ideal scenario she created where she had the best of both worlds being a mom and working woman. I admire that she will do anything for her kids. She goes to such extremes to help Micah and me that people joke about things that are "so Diane." I also admire that she was able to maintain her career and keep her work separate and her clients happy even when we as a family were going through really hard times with my health. And she has a great relationship with *her* mom.

She is a role model in many ways.

I have followed in her footsteps work-wise so far, sort of forging a nontraditional career path that involves writing and freelancing for multiple clients. I think I've also modeled my life after hers in ways I'm not really conscious of. People tell us we're similar, but in some ways we're radically different.

I decided to take another path in terms of the pace of life. I think it's important to "stop and smell the roses," whereas she just charges through life at a constant fast pace.

She did give me the best advice: Find the joy in every day. That was a good one. I've adopted the mantra "Live Happy."

My mom had lots of behaviors that growing up I said I would NEVER do when I got older. I should have written them down because now I can't remember what they are. (Seeing the past with rose-colored glasses, I guess.)

Her advice for the twenties: Establish roots (has really swayed me against traveling). Create a community (makes me more inclined to pursue and maintain friendships). Take dating seriously so you don't turn thirty and wish you were married. Live healthy.

Most important to who I am today: she taught me to prioritize love over all else.

My mom has been a huge part of my life and always will be. I think my job now as an adult is to establish boundaries, and, in a way, moving to San Francisco is the best thing I could have done. Forced to move into my own apartment that's not a thirty-minute drive from my parents' house . . . so important. I already feel like I can breathe (figuratively), it's more spacious, I'm more relaxed. When I wake up, the day is mine to take charge of and do what I want with it. I get to determine the course of my days, which determines the course of my weeks, which determines ultimately whether I have a life I'm proud of. And when I was living in L.A. last year I wasn't living a life I was proud of . . . I look back on that year and I'm like what did I accomplish? How did I grow as a person? Obviously, all the hospitalizations were a challenge, but even before that I feel like I was just regressing from spending so much time at home and allowing my parents to help me as much as they did.

But I don't hold any of this against my mom anymore. I used to. A letter I wrote to her in 2008 reveals how mad I was:

> When I do my treatment is not up to you. If I choose to do it before I go out, I will do it before. If I choose to do it after, I will do it after. It is my decision. Stop treating me like a child and trying to make choices for me. It is not your right or your duty as a parent to do that; your duty as a parent is to support and guide the decisions that I make.
>
> You may calmly suggest, if you wish, that I do treatments by a certain time, but that does not by any means mean that I must do so. You decide to go to sleep when you are tired; I get to decide when I go to sleep. If you don't like me coming home late and doing treatment, try to remember this: if you don't allow me to go out, I can sneak out. It is impossible for you to force me to do something against my will. I have always been a good kid, I tell you where I'm going and what I'm doing. However, you seem to not trust my judgment. You seem to think you know what's best for me better than I do. But you don't.

I realize that now that I'm an adult it's my job, not hers, to establish my independence and autonomy. Perhaps she didn't do the best job in certain ways of setting me up to be a successful adult. But she was also worried that I wasn't going to live long so I understand why my independence wasn't her top priority. She just wanted me to live. If I do have kids, a lot of the issues I faced with my mom won't be relevant, since I won't have a kid with CF.

4/28/16

I remember the time I went to Bed Bath & Beyond and stood next to Jamie Lee Curtis while picking out a duffel bag for sleepaway camp. She asked if I was shopping to go off to college. It amused me that people thought I was years older than I actually was; I didn't realize how unusual that is for a CF patient, that most other kids with CF look many years younger than they are. Despite what everyone said—that I would love being tall one day, that they would steal inches off my legs if they could—I wanted to be short. I quite literally would fall asleep at night fantasizing that I'd wake up short. Those critical years I spent hunched over, made worse by a lifetime of coughing, still reveal themselves in my rounded posture today.

I did not have any friends with CF growing up, and thus had no concept of the roller-coaster of illness patients ride, at varying velocities. Waddington's "epigenetic landscape" model, which I first learned about in human biology classes in college, gives me a framework to understand the way we with CF both can and cannot control our futures. Epigenetics refers to the study of how DNA (your genes) can be modified based on inputs from the environment; genes are regulated structurally and chemically, turned on or off by processes like phosphorylation* or methylation.** Basically, the epigenetic landscape is a hill that marbles can roll down. Your genes dictate the range of possible endpoints the marbles can roll to, but epigenetic modification determines which endpoint the marble actually falls on.

With cystic fibrosis, I believe our genes determine the various possibilities for the trajectory of illness: how fast our lung function

---

* a biochemical process that involves the addition of phosphate to an organic compound

** a process by which methyl groups are added to the DNA molecule

will deteriorate, how likely our lungs are to be colonized by op-portunistic pathogens, whether our lungs or our pancreas or our liver will be the most affected organ. But within that range of possibilities, environmental factors like access to good healthcare, age of diagnosis, where we live, what family we're born into, and random chance all contribute to determining our health out-comes. I conceptualize it like this: our genes dictate the endpoint; our choices, environment, and chance dictate how fast we get there and the rockiness of the descent.

My CF friendships started in the hospital, in walks with masks on and in time spent sitting outside by the fountain six feet apart. To this day, I maintain them through texting, phones, and social media. Having friends with my same disease satisfied my desire for something I didn't even realize I'd wanted: a confidante, some-one who understood exactly what I live with day to day. My CF friends have offered strength, resilience, and unwavering support to help pull me through the toughest times. Before Melissa went on life support, lived in the ICU for nearly a month, and then had a successful lung transplant, we were talking nearly every day over text while we both did our vest and nebulizer treatments. Now, she's slowly recovering from her lung transplant. Another friend with CF died in late August last year, shattering my world and forcing me to pick up the pieces while simultaneously battling my own wildly unstable health. When I found out, I didn't sleep for days; at night, I would get out of bed, seeking a distraction from grief, and lie on the kitchen floor with Kona, listening to music.

The range of disease trajectories is huge—from people who need transplants as teenagers to people who are in their twenties with 90 percent lung function. It puts into perspective where I am on the spectrum, where it's likely I'll go, and how fast. It's troubling to see someone once healthier than me either die or progress to end-stage disease. Beyond the bone-deep ache and grief I feel for their families, I preemptively ache and grieve for mine, knowing that one day they will probably have to bury me.

People have always called me an inspiration, but I'm not. I do sweat the small stuff, just like everyone else. I just happen to also have to sweat the big, life-or-death stuff. The burden of being an inspiration is heavy, because it means you have to be positive all the time, no matter what you're going through.

It reminds me of the Stanford Duck Syndrome. Despite its cutesy name, it's no fucking joke. Here's the idea: At Stanford, students are like ducks gliding on the water. On the surface, when ducks move, no one sees their legs below the water, paddling furiously to stay afloat. Students at Stanford, from the outside, are the image of perfection; they're able to maintain straight As, intimidating résumés, and a laundry list of extracurriculars while simultaneously finding time to eat well, exercise, party, see friends, travel, and look good. All the while *it's supposed to look easy.* Mental health issues are taboo among the student body; since everyone else seems like they're effortlessly getting by, each person struggling with their mental health feels alone. It's a vicious cycle of silence and struggle, which has driven some to suicide.

The Duck Syndrome is a dangerous phenomenon that is not quarantined to Stanford's campus—I find the same patterns all over sunny California, and despite having left Stanford over a year ago, I still find myself refusing to let anyone peer below the surface and see me furiously paddling to stay afloat when I'm going through a rough time. I want to work on that, acknowledge the ups and downs in life in a way that's devoid of self-pity and respectful of the fact that things could always be worse.

For me to be an inspiration, the expectation is that I glide, like a duck defying physics. That is what we want to see, because it gives us hope that it's what we ourselves can achieve. But when I'm in the ER and in the midst of an acute health crisis, I'm not happily greeting every single person who comes to poke and prod. I'm not thanking any sort of God for the thousands of things I have to be grateful for. When I'm really struggling to breathe, I'm not saying, "Well, I have pneumonia for the third time in two months, but at least I have all my limbs!" Sometimes I have moments when I'm very sick and also very grateful, but other times, I wallow in self-pity temporarily before I rise above it and tackle the next obstacle in my way.

I discovered that as a sophomore in college. That year was the toughest until that point, with many months spent in the hospital and on IVs and dozens of new complications. One day, I walked out of the triple I shared with Maya and Makiko and went across the hall to the lounge of my dorm, where I lay under the table and sobbed (being underneath tables on the floor is strangely comforting to me in crisis moments). After I was done, I headed to the ER to deal with the current crisis, but I was better able to face it having dealt with my own negative emotions and fears first.

I've found that such is the task of a writer: to help others understand and empathize with a life experience they've never lived. Work hard at empathy, and two things will happen: First, you will feel better about your existence. Second, you will find that you're not so alone after all, and that there's always somewhere to turn to, even if it's just the blank page and the blinking cursor.

I don't want constant, unwavering happiness. Now, I want perspective. I don't want to numb the experience of pain. I want to be resilient.

I'm not an inspiration. I'm just a person, grounded in compassion, striving to achieve empathy and wanting to make my way with goodness and grace.

5/3/16

Whenever it happens, I wonder, "Will this be the time?"

Will this be the time when the blood spilling up my lungs and out my mouth will burst forth so fast that I can't breathe? The time when I'll be passed out on the floor from blood loss by the time the ambulance arrives? The time my hemoptysis isn't just a scare, but the final, swift, deadly bullet?

This isn't an entirely unlikely scenario. It's the scene that flashes for an instant through my mind whenever I cough up frank red blood in bigger-than-tiny quantities. It's the end my doctor has warned me about for years. Each time it happens, as I cough and cough and wait for the bleeding to subside, my lips a bold Marilyn Monroe red, I'm not scared—it's too common. But it occurs to me that maybe I should be. Because each time could be *that* time.

The locations where it's happened have been diverse and darkly amusing: On my high school's front lawn as we ate lunch. In the locker room of a Burton store, unclothed but for one leg stuck in a wetsuit. In the ocean, while surfing. In a backyard, playing spike ball. Lying in bed, awakened from sleep. At my high school after-prom party. At a concert, lungs irritated from second-hand smoke. At volleyball tournaments. At water polo tournaments. At swim meets. In yoga classes. In my parents' house. In my own apartment, completely alone. In front of strangers as I sat on the curb in front of my family's favorite steak house. On a bench at the gym, with terrified onlookers. In a plane going across the Pacific Ocean, where all I could do was hope it would stop. On hikes in Hawaii. In a swimming pool. Mid-kiss. The list could go on.

Often, the comically absurd nature of my parade of hemoptysis-through-random-and-amusing-locations distracts me from fear. I can laugh about it, especially when it's over and I'm in the clear. But when I reflect back on all these times, it's rattling to realize just how many times I could have died had the bleeds not stopped. It feels like luck's been on my side, and odds are that won't be true forever.

How do we live with the impending fear of a deadly event? I've noticed that as my hemoptysis has worsened, I've almost displaced my fear of death onto other, extremely unlikely situations: shark attacks, plane crashes, car accidents, abductions, armed robberies, and other subjects of a paranoid person's nightmares. Things that never scared me before now terrify me. But simultaneously, in the moment, hemoptysis events that actually could be deadly do not scare me. I can't psychoanalyze that, but I'm sure someone can.

5/8/16

Thinking of my mom as we celebrate Mother's Day. I am one of the lucky ones, to have scored a family like mine. I won the lottery.

My selfless mom has spent twenty-three years trying to give me the best life possible: bringing cookies and pasta to every volleyball or water polo game or swim meet in high school; flying up to Northern California to take care of me whenever I was sick in college; encouraging me to pursue my love of sports and the ocean no matter how hard it became; and my personal favorite, embarrassing me for years on end by honking to indicate CBAs (Cute Boy Alerts).

To be a mother is hard enough without added complications. To be a mother to a kid with a condition you're told is terminal, and to make that kid's life incredible and fun and filled with awe and surprise anyway, is miracle work. Beyond that, not everyone can say their mother is their Wingmom, but anyone who knows my mom will attest that she's the best of the best. She's a force—

beyond her dual jobs caring for Micah and me, and working in PR and marketing, she has managed to mobilize our community and raise over $3 million for CF research since I was diagnosed.

My mom is my rock. Simply put, I don't know what I'd do without her. And she learned how to be a mom from her own mom, my grandma, who is the coolest grandma out there.

5/20/16

Wednesday I went to clinic and Dr. Mohabir decided to take me off IVs! I was stunned and ecstatic. That's an understatement. I can't remember feeling happier in recent history. I was elated. Stoked. Beyond shocked. It was so unexpected. I left the clinic, it was sunny out, I discontinued my meropenem drip, went to Aunt Lissa's, did some work, and then pulled out my own port (so nice that I can do that with the port, as opposed to the PICC, which someone else has to remove).

Friday I had a phone interview for a writing job at Tribe Dynamics. I explained to them that I would have to be part-time. And we talked for thirty minutes, then they said if they decided they wanted to proceed, they'd give me a writing and editing assignment as the next step, which they did! I was so happy. Very good for my ego and self-confidence as a writer.

PART FOUR

When Mal wasn't well enough to practice in the pool, her mom would often ask me to take her out for walks around the neighborhood just to get her heart pumping and, as Diane would say, "get the mucus moving." To me it seemed like that was the extent of it, a nagging case of bronchitis or maybe just a little pesky congestion that needed to be shaken loose. Then on one of these walks Mal started coughing. A lot. I remembered that Diane was always encouraging her to cough up, so I thought, "Hey, this walking is really helping!" And I pushed her to continue. Then Mal showed me the blood. She didn't seem all that concerned—and even managed a couple of embarrassed yet composed giggles. I was frozen and felt at that moment like I was the child and she was the adult looking after me.

—COACH ROB BOWIE

5/22/16

So much on my mind right now.

The past week was amazing, stressful, challenging, exciting, worrisome, busy, anxious, fun. SOOOO fun.

Tuesday morning I got ready and drove to Pacifica to meet Jack for our first date to go surfing. We met on New Year's Eve at Ali's pregame before we went to the Snapchat company party but didn't see each other again until a few months later when I moved up here. His friend Justin is my roommate's boyfriend. Ari organized a brunch and invited me. I sat next to Jack. He's smart, cute, cool.

We met at Nor Cal Surf Shop, rented boards and wetsuits, and went down to the beach. In the water, he was so sweet, almost protective, pushing me when my arms got tired, making sure I was safe and could catch my breath, etc. There was this moment when I was looking at the houses on the hillside and talking about how beautiful they were and saying how nice it would be to just live there and write and look at the beach and take surf breaks and then go back and write more. And he was looking at me while I was talking about that and it made me feel as if he really liked me. Or maybe he was just attracted to me.

He caught a couple of waves. My arms were like lead. I needed all the pushes I could get just to paddle out and stay out of the impact zone. Finally when a good wave rolled around for me, he pushed me and I took it. It wasn't a great ride, the wave died out on me once I stood up, but it was nice to see that at least popping up still felt natural. I didn't lose that (even if I've lost all of my paddling strength).

After that ride, he caught a wave in so he could help me paddle back out, but it was bad timing, with a big set rolling through. I couldn't catch my breath since I kept having to turtle, wave after wave. We ended up just paddling in to rest and sat on the beach for a bit. We got onto the sand, and I sat down on my board and he sat down next to me on mine instead of sitting on his. We were chatting for a little, then he asked about my LXV tattoo, and I told him that it was sixty-five, for sixty-five roses, the nickname for cystic fibrosis. And when I was done, he looked at me for a second and said, "You are so beautiful," and I said thank you, and he leaned in and kissed me. I kissed him back.

For the rest of the afternoon, Jack and I hung out on the beach, lay in the sun, kissed, chatted, etc. It was lovely, the first beach/surf day I've had in so long, and the first time I'd kissed anyone in a very long time. I was so shocked by how the day developed, like it wasn't reality. I just never ever expected that would happen; even though I kind of suspected that he was into me or attracted to me, I really didn't think he would just make a move on me like that, especially in broad daylight, especially so soon. It made me happy.

This week I also had to do the writing assignment for the Tribe Dynamics job, which was a really difficult assignment since I have no experience in marketing. The editing portion was easy, actually, but the research/writing was hard. I have no idea if I did what I was supposed to do, but I worked hard, so if I don't get the job, it probably means I wasn't the right fit for it. Now that I've turned in the assignment, I'm not stressed about it, but I was super stressed while working on it. I also had articles to write and a chapter for Susan's book plus a creative nonfiction piece for a blog Natalie wants to create. So work has been nutty, but rewarding and interesting. After this week I feel proud of myself for my versatility and progress as a writer.

Friday was such a crazy day. I got home at like 9:00 p.m. after ten hours out of the house. I still had to do treatment.

The next night I had another date with Jack that went really well. The museum we went to was a bit strange but very interesting, and he was fun to hang out with. It felt very, very couple-y. After the museum we went to a restaurant about a fifteen-minute walk away, a little French place. We both got burgers and cocktails. It was delicious and we had a lot of fun. He said he was thinking about coming down to L.A. to hang out with me before going to San Diego to see his mom. I said I thought it was a great idea. He said he didn't want to put any pressure on things or make things weird (by meeting my family). I said it would be great.

Jack says he wants to take things slowly, I think basically to establish that there's more to us than attraction. That's the reason he planned a whole date near the Caltrain station, so he wouldn't be tempted to come back and stay over at my place. I told him I respected that and was fine with taking things slowly. It seemed early to leave the city at 8:15, but given what he said about taking things slow, it made sense. I like how we're honest with each other and communicative because I feel like I know what's going on.

6/1/16

Memorial Day weekend I got to go home and see my family and friends! My plan had been to surf every day while at home, but I had fevers and learned the hard way that surfing with a fever and shortness of breath is dangerous. I asked myself the questions that come up each time I'm struck with my four classic sickness symptoms (shortness of breath, fatigue, fever, and hemoptysis): Do I need to call Stanford? Do I need to go to the ER now? Not wanting to get stuck admitted at a hospital in L.A. with an order from Stanford doctors not to fly back north,

I didn't call anyone and got through the week. I had a secondary motive to hide symptoms—I wanted to see my friends Alex and Hannah become Mr. and Mrs. Rosenthal that weekend, the original reason for my trip to L.A. and a wedding I would have been devastated to miss.

Jack came to L.A. that next weekend and met my parents and grandparents!

I made it through the week, went to the wedding, happily dancing and celebrating the newlyweds as long as I could before needing to sit down and enjoy the night from my seat. Later that night, my fever spiked, and I knew that I would be admitted and go back on IV antibiotics as soon as I got back up north. I tossed and turned all night, hoping that I wasn't sabotaging my own body by not going to the emergency room right then.

6/10/16

With a burgeoning relationship, I wonder how much to divulge to Jack about the possibility that dire things could happen to me, and my fears that they will. My physical fragility and my underlying emotional anxiety. Will he run away? Will he view me as too fragile and stop seeing me as an equal, a partner? Will he want to go the long course with someone who might not be able to make it to the finish line? Or will he make up some excuse and duck out once he realizes the reality of this fucked-up, shitty, relentless, unforgiving, merciless disease?

The other thing on my mind right now is travel. We have a trip to Vegas planned in just about a month now. We're going to be flying together early Friday afternoon and coming back late Sunday night. With how my GI problems have been and my own irrational fear of exposing GI issues to a significant other (the details at least), I'm terrified at the idea of sharing a hotel room and having no privacy. I'm worried I won't sleep, I'm worried that if

I'm not already sick when I go, it's 100 percent inevitable that I will leave sick. I worry about the fact that I can't just plan a trip to Vegas with a new boyfriend (I think that's what he is) and be excited about it. I wonder if I will ever be able to plan trips and feel excited again, or if I will always have anxieties, especially these particular ones that I don't feel capable of discussing with anyone (other than my parents). Can I send him off to breakfast with the other people and stay in the room and do treatment/go to the bathroom in privacy? I just don't see him wanting to leave me and go with other people. He also brought up the fact that toward the end of summer, he's going to his family's lake house property in Maine, and that he was thinking of inviting me and another couple. It's terrifying, but I'm so happy that he wants me to come.

6/12/16

On June 8, when I saw my Stanford doctors, I reentered the hospital and resumed the same IV and oral antibiotic regimen I had discontinued just four weeks prior. We planned for three to six weeks on the course, and a few days later, after some improvement in my clinical symptoms, the doctors discharged me and allowed me to go home on home therapy. The drugs began to work, and again, I felt a wave of relief wash over me as I resumed my daily routine of work, treatments, exercise, and evening plans with friends.

But after a week, I began to decline again, and found myself struggling with the fateful four harbingers of a pulmonary exacerbation. This time was different, though—I was already on IVs. How could I be getting worse while on antibiotic therapy? What could I be doing differently? I stayed home all week, cooked the most nutritious foods I could think of, slept a ton, and did extra treatments, but still, the symptoms persisted.

6/19/16

It's Father's Day so I'm thinking about my dad. He's amazing—the one responsible for my intellectual curiosity and my philosophical musings, he's driven thousands of miles on road trips with me (with many Denny's stops along the way), he's spent hundreds of nights on a chair or cot at my bedside in the hospital, he selflessly puts his family before himself no matter what. He's my own personal lawyer, fighting to get me every drug my insurance company tries to deny.

7/5/16

By the time I went to clinic, I knew my lung function would be down (it was, by almost 10 percent) and that the doctors would want to admit me again to change the plan. Being mentally prepared for an admission helps. My bag was filled with snacks, a phone charger, my laptop, a book, extra underwear, a toothbrush, and certain medications I need that the hospital doesn't carry. I walked from clinic to the admitting desk, signed papers to appoint my mom and dad as the decision makers for me if I were to become incapacitated, and ate dinner in the cafeteria.

Walking down the hallway to my room in the B1 wing, I greeted familiar faces that I hadn't seen since I graduated college in December 2014—my last admission in B1 was my last week of my last quarter at Stanford. Expecting a hospitalization has a strange way of making it feel normal, even though being hospitalized four times in six months at my age is so, so far from normal.

Now, I'm still on B1, on day 6 of this admission. Not a whole lot has changed—I lost the fevers but gained terrible chest pain, improved a little, then got a little worse again. When I'm not walking laps around the fountain in front, IV pole in tow, I'm receiving oxygen in my nasal cannula to ease the shortness of breath and headaches. Visits make the time go by, and I'm so thankful for that. Little things like Philz coffee deliveries and fresh peaches in the cafeteria make my day. Life goes on, with work deadlines still demanding attention.

In so many ways, life in the hospital is like life on the outside. For the most part, my mind focuses on the present moment—my current treatment, my step count, chatting with friends, hanging out with my mom, reading a good book, getting work done, enjoying the sunshine sitting out by the fountain with my feet in the water. It can be easy to forget that I'm receiving big doses of powerful medications that could, one day, stop working entirely.

But then there are times that remind me of the magnitude of the situation, of the fact that these little daily/weekly/monthly challenges—and whether I win or lose at them—could determine my life span. Today I blew as hard as I could on my lung function test, and when I saw no improvement from the week before despite four weeks of continuous IVs, a week of hospitalization, and new antibiotics on board, I wondered briefly whether all this fighting is pointless. Will it make a difference which antibiotics we use, or are they all ineffective? Will this disease ultimately do what it wants with me regardless of the weapons we throw at it, laughing at our attempts to keep infection at bay?

If a wave holds you under for too long while you're out surfing, the worst thing you can do is struggle and fight against the water; when drowning and in danger, the best chance you have is to try to relax, hold your breath, and wait until you're given the chance to pop to the surface. Sometimes acceptance and ease, rather than force and struggle, are the keys to survival.

A few hours after my lung function test today, one of the medical providers brought up for the first time the idea of placing a feeding tube. Most of the time, with CF, routines are familiar, and the pace of change with the medical regimen is slow—add a pill here, subtract a pill there, add some IVs, undergo some hospitalizations. All of that is very familiar. But when we get a new diagnosis, we have to make sense of a whole new series of reductions in quality of life. When I was found to have multiple pulmonary emboli in my lungs and had to start blood thinners was one of those times. When my hemoptysis first began to worsen, and I had to reimagine a life never lived more than an hour from a major medical center was another one of those times.

Having to get a feeding tube, which would add complexity to my regimen and force me to cede control over another aspect of my life, would also be one of those times. The news was startling, as I look very healthy and am at a healthy weight. I told her: *I want to wait to do that until I really really need it, and I'm just not there yet.* But the provider explained that oftentimes, patients wait too long to get a feeding tube placed, until they "really really need it," and by then, it's too late—their respiratory status has declined to the point where surgery to implant the tube is no longer safe. Her explanation was informed by the knowledge and expertise she's gained working with hundreds of patients, whereas my interpretation of the wisdom of my getting a feeding tube was informed only by my own clinical history and an aversion to discomfort.

One of the difficulties with CF is that progressive decline is inevitable, but the rate at which the decline will happen is unpredictable. I could have five good years left with relatively stable lung function and weight. I could even have ten or fifteen or twenty good years. Or, my infection could rapidly worsen, my lung function and weight could both plummet, and at that point, this provider would be right, it would be too late to place a feeding tube. As patients, we have to make decisions balancing two often-disparate goals—maintaining current quality of life while extending life span—without complete information about how much threat we're really facing. I don't want to diminish my quality of life too early, but I don't want to wait so long that getting the treatment I need isn't possible.

I recently finished a book by the late neurosurgeon Paul Kalanithi, *When Breath Becomes Air.* After working his entire life to become a neurosurgeon and ending up a chief resident at Stanford, he was hit with a diagnosis of stage IV lung cancer. His career path had been brimming with opportunity—to become a renowned neurosurgeon/neuroscientist, to do research that would change lives, and to continue operating on the very organ that makes people who they are. And then in a blink, everything shifted.

The life he had been leading was gone. The diagnosis left him facing his mortality at a much younger age than he ever thought he would have to. It forced him to consider the question of what makes life meaningful—which had long held his interest in an abstract sense—in a concrete, urgent, and highly personal way.

Lung cancer and cystic fibrosis are very different illnesses, of course, but throughout the book I found myself laughing, crying, highlighting, underlining, and saying yes, yes, yes, yes, yes. So much of it resonated.

With his diagnosis shining a spotlight on his mortality, he wondered how he should spend his time. "The way forward would seem obvious," he wrote, "if only I knew how many months or years I had left. Tell me three months, I'd spend time with family. Tell me one year, I'd write a book. Give me ten years, I'd get back to treating diseases. The truth that you live one day at a time didn't help: What was I supposed to do with that day?"

The question of how to meaningfully spend a life is not unique to those of us with health challenges. None of us knows if our life will be cut short. But for people with cystic fibrosis, or stage IV lung cancer, or any other life-limiting illness, there is a certainty that life will most likely be cut short to some extent.

This certainty forces us to examine our values, prioritize our time, and search for meaning now rather than later. "I began to realize that coming in such close contact with my own mortality had changed both nothing and everything," Kalanithi wrote. "Before my cancer was diagnosed, I knew that someday I would die, but I didn't know when. After the diagnosis, I knew that someday I would die, but I didn't know when. But now I knew it acutely."

Kalanithi hits the nail on the head of one of the more frustrating aspects of trying to make the most of whatever amount of time we may have. "The most obvious might be an impulse to frantic activity: to 'live life to its fullest,' to travel, to dine, to achieve a host of neglected ambitions. Part of the cruelty of cancer, though, is not only that it limits your time; it also limits your energy, vastly reducing the amount you can squeeze into a day. . . . Some days, I simply persist." Some days, I simply persist; some days, I simply breathe.

A few weeks ago, on a night when I wasn't sure how to keep managing it all, I finished Paul Kalanithi's book and cried. But it reminded me of the way to move forward, the way I've been operating my entire life: "Maybe, in the absence of any certainty, we should just assume that we're going to live a long time. Maybe that's the only way forward. . . . Even if I'm dying, until I actually die, I am still living."

7/11/16
They told me I was resistant to all of the antibiotics. They brought the infectious disease doctors on board and overall the outlook was very bleak. My oxygen was low so I was wearing the cannula, and I was having trouble walking. I started having chest pain. My GI was not good. My weight went down to 139.

But then they switched me to Ceptaz/avibactam instead of just Ceptaz, and put me on TOBI instead of colistin. A little while later they switched me to IV Bactrim instead of oral (at my urging), because the oral makes me more nauseous but probably works better. They also added oral minocycline. Day after day, nothing was really happening, I wasn't really improving.

But then I started to turn around and got discharged the next Thursday, day 8. One thing during this hospitalization made me happy . . . Jack came to visit every day from Thursday to Monday. Then he got busy with school.

I'm scared the IVs aren't going to work anymore. They keep me on them even though I'm resistant to each one. The theory is that synergistically they provide some help. I just want to make it to Hawaii on August 19 with my parents, Micah, Jack, Matt, and Michelle. Haven't been to Maui in a year and I miss the sun and the warm ocean so so so much. It's painful to think about how much I miss it.

Caleigh went to Hawaii for two weeks and had the time of her life and then the day I got admitted, her mom called me from there to ask the name of the hospital I was admitted to. Caleigh had a bad bowel blockage and needed surgery but they couldn't do it there because she's too complicated. She was in so much pain. She ended up on a ventilator because she couldn't breathe, she got pneumonia, and they medevacked her to Stanford's ICU and it was heartbreaking that there was nothing we could do to help. Melissa and Emily★ were both checking in with me about both my health and Caleigh's. I had more info about her since her mom was updating my mom and me.

I kept picturing her in the ICU, unconscious, unable to

★ another friend with CF and the founder of Emily's Entourage

breathe without life support, going on ECMO,* her family watching her like that, her dad and sister flying in to be with them, unable to do anything. How could they manage, how could they hold it together? How would my family deal with that? What would I want if I were in her circumstances? Or, better put, what *will* I want *when I am* in her circumstances? Because one day it will happen, that is inevitable. The when is unclear, but the fact that one day it will happen seems inevitable.

Since my *cepacia* is resistant to antibiotics, the stakes are higher, and I'm starting to see myself in Caleigh. How ironic that the writing I've been doing for Nelson Hardiman about California's death with dignity law will be relevant to my life one day soon, if I end up on a vent or suffering in some extreme way and am not able to get a lung transplant because of the *cepacia*.

7/19/16

The last two days have been madness. I've had a million things to do all at once—we're in the final throes for Susan's book, writing for Nelson Hardiman, writing for Janet,** editing an app for a friend, editing Dr. David Weill's memoir about running a transplant program, writing a blog post for *Emily's Entourage*.

The more time we spend together, the more I feel myself falling for Jack. In the beginning I wasn't sure if we had a connection other than physical attraction, but I don't feel that way anymore. I appreciate that he feels like he can talk to me about anything, and I think I'm getting to the point where I feel more comfortable talking to him about more important things.

I'm really excited about Hawaii, which is only a month away!

---

* Similar to the heart-lung bypass machine used in open-heart surgery. It pumps and oxygenates a patient's blood outside the body, allowing the heart and lungs to rest.
** the founder and curator of ArtHealingArtists

7/21/16

My GI issues have once again taken over my life. This is how it was in my senior year of college. I remember having a tormented relationship with food, constantly being hungry but also being afraid to eat; then eating anyway, never knowing how much to eat or what foods would be good or bad for my stomach. I had horrible body image and self-loathing issues for not having a body that functions properly.

Things with my GI are as bad now as they ever were. I need to get a handle on it and wish Dr. Mohabir would let me try ataluren again because I can't fucking deal with it anymore.

Getting the infection under control feels beyond my control. They extended my IV regimen instead of taking me off IVs or admitting me. They put me back on the same regimen I'd been on three weeks before, the one that I got sick on. I need a punching bag. . . .

I don't really feel like I have an outlet for this and I have so much anger right now. I can't talk to my parents about this or they'll force me into therapy. As I get older, the more I realize how hard my disease must be for them and how much fear they must have, too, the more I don't want to dump my anger on them. I want to be strong for them, or at least pretend to be strong. I can't talk to my friends because they won't understand. And not Jack for sure because I'm not comfortable even acknowledging that I have GI problems.

I remember asking Kari about how she discussed the topic with her then boyfriend (now husband), Brad. She said she had to tell him something, and just told him straight up what she struggles with. Apparently he said, "That's what you were so scared to tell me?" And she said something like, "But don't you find it disgusting?" And he basically said something like, "You're beautiful to me no matter what." He loved her unconditionally.

I just spent a solid twenty minutes reading old conversations between Kari and me on Facebook Messenger from 2014. Back then, I was still planning to live in New Zealand after graduation. And she was still alive. So much has changed. She was worrying about internships and job applications then. I was trying to figure out my postcollege plans and career goals. I admired that she was so dedicated to working despite her health status; who knew she would be dead a year later? We were both admitted at the same time for GI stuff, both dealing with dehumanizing enemas and communication issues with the team, both wondering about the best way to disclose CF in the workplace, to friends, to boyfriends. So many of the same issues I still think about now, except I'm still here to ponder them and she's not.

My ability to talk to others with CF has waned a little bit. The main three that I always kept in touch with were Melissa, Kari, and Caleigh. But things are so different now with Melissa and Caleigh having had their transplants and Kari being gone. Melissa and Caleigh both could have died a number of times; fundamentally, they've been through things I cannot understand and have every reason to fear. They reached the end of the CF spectrum and jumped onto a completely different one—the transplant spectrum. Their lives are so different and their health status is incomprehensible to me now: I don't know the intricacies of life post-transplant, and for them, the troubles of life as a CF patient with 40 to 50 percent lung function are in the distant past. I don't think we relate in the same way anymore. I find myself not knowing what to say, thrust into the position that probably most of my friends and acquaintances are in when they hear about my health. When I try to talk to Melissa and Caleigh, I feel uncomfortable, wanting to say just the right thing but having no idea what that right thing is and fumbling with words. Melissa and Caleigh always listen when I have complaining to do, but I don't feel right about it given what they've been through. They've been at death's door, they've been on ventilators, they've had their families crying beside them, wondering if they'll make it through the night. They've had their chests ripped open, their old lungs torn out and new ones placed in, like magic, except it's not magic and there seem to be as many problems post-transplant as there were before.

7/23/16
The day after I wrote that last post I started to feel much better emotionally.

Last Friday, Jack came to the city to have dinner with my parents and Glen and Sandra, which was truly a hilarious event. He knows nothing about Judaism and it was a Shabbat dinner, so he got a full-on Jewish education, learning about the kiddush cup, the prayers, what a Seder is, the story of Passover, what a *kippah* is, etc. Sandra gave him a lot of shit and he was taking it well— apparently, she liked him a lot.

After we got home that night, we talked for a really long time about so many things. In this relationship, I'm scared I'm the one who's going to get hurt, for two reasons: 1) I wonder if part of him still has feelings for his old girlfriend and 2) in December, he's going to move wherever he needs to be for his career, and that might not be S.F. And even if it is S.F., if he ultimately plans to move to the East Coast, I'm going to have to think long and hard about whether to spend so much time in a relationship with someone who probably can't be with me long-term.

For now, though, things are really good. We debriefed the dinner and laughed a lot. I like that he's so willing to spend time with my parents and family. I think Jack values family a lot. I wonder if I will meet his mom at some point? She doesn't seem to come up here often but I know they are very close. He's going on a trip with her to Oregon in September and we're still discussing the possibility of me going to Maine with him and his dad, which I keep going back and forth about.

PART FIVE

It is not every day that you run into an individual that is far older and wiser than her stated age. Mallory leaves behind a message to be remembered. Facing the unconquerable with perseverance, determination, and realism is a victory even in the face of death. Mal gives all patients with cystic fibrosis the hope of survival and the possibility that you can Live Happy with chronic illness. Mallory has taught me that although I have suffered her loss, I have gained a story of love to be told. A love of her, a love of hope, and a love of life, which lead many of us on the path to find a cure.

—Paul Mohabir,
Director of the Adult CF Program
at Stanford University Hospital

7/28/16

So much has changed in just the last few days.

Over the weekend, I started to feel more short of breath but went hiking at Lands End anyway (probably was overkill). It was a really nice day, but too intense, cardio-wise. Monday, I woke up feeling way worse. Luckily my mom was visiting, and just as we were about to pull up to the house after running errands, I felt a bleed coming on.

7/29/16

. . . continuing where I left off last night.

My mom pulled over on the side of the road because I told her blood was coming and I didn't want to splatter it all over the car. I grabbed a pill bottle that was inside the cup holder in between the two front seats, dumped the pills out, and started coughing the blood in there. I got myself onto the curb and the blood kept coming—at 20 ccs, it was big enough and unexpected enough to be scary.

Right then, a woman from AffloVest drove up, bringing my new portable vest, something I've been wanting for five years. It was finally here, and I was bent over coughing blood on the street, too exhausted, feverish, and distracted to focus on this life-altering machine.

When the bleeding stopped, we went inside and she showed me how to set the vest up. I was shivering so I put on my fever scarf—the striped one from the Gap I got so many years ago. Hot tea, a big jacket, my scarf, chills—the telltale signs of fever. I checked my temp and it was 102.3, high but not crazy high.

My mom and I got into a fight over whether to call the fellow. She sometimes thinks fellows say to come in to the hospital to cover their asses—they don't want to get sued if you don't go to the ER and something goes wrong.

My thinking is, if there's a protocol that says hemoptysis + fever + multidrug-resistant bacteria + shortness of breath = a trip to the ER, then you follow it. Because even if nine out of ten times it wouldn't matter if you waited the twelve hours until morning to go to the hospital, there's the one time it might make the difference between life and death.

We struck a compromise and told the fellow on call that if he could get Dr. Chhatwani from Stanford's CF team on the phone, we would do what she said. The fellow called us back and said he reached her and that Dr. C wanted me to go to the ER so I immediately packed my bags. I texted Jack to tell him about the hemoptysis and about the ER visit, and he called and offered to come, which was so thoughtful. He scored a lot of points with that offer.

The night was uneventful. The ER part went smoothly because I had brought my nighttime IVs from home and I got up to my own room at about 1:00 a.m. I was so exhausted, feverish, and short of breath by that point that I could barely keep my eyes open while they did the admission and asked me all the same questions I answer every single time.

The repetition of things can be comforting, and it can be infuriating. The fact that things are familiar is what's comforting. But having to go over my belongings list every single time I'm admitted and having to do it not only in the ER but also again in the room is ridiculous. Having to go through every single medication is a little annoying but not ridiculous. Having to repeat the tests in the room that they already ran in the ER is frustrating and creates unnecessary expense, plus it means I don't get to sleep.

My white count was 22,000, so very high. Not surprising given the fever and how I felt. They took blood cultures, but so far nothing has come back.

I didn't realize how concerned the docs were when I first got here. I was highly concerned that I had gone down to a lesser IV regimen at home the week before, when I was already unwell, and then got sicker. I began to worry about whether the drugs would be able to get this under control. It seemed like, after getting sick so many times in a row while on IVs, with few changes to the regimen, there was little else they could try.

The next morning, we saw Dr. Chhatwani and the whole CF team. They explained how serious this was and said they were going to reach beyond Stanford's infectious disease team to *cepacia* specialists at other centers (like Toronto), and that they were going to try new things. And they did!

The next blood draw showed my white count at 17,000. A little movement in the right direction, but I was still having really high fevers. Today is the first day I don't have a high fever—the highest today has been 100.6. I've felt hot and clammy all evening but at least I'm not in the 102s. That's reassuring.

Wednesday I'm sitting in my room with Coach Bowie, who had come to visit. We had a nice chat, reminiscing about high school water polo days, then he went with my mom to the cafeteria and they were gonna get food and bring it back to eat in the room. While they were gone, I heard a distinctive knock but didn't put two and two together to recognize Dr. Mohabir's knock because he'd been on some sort of leave for months. He bounded in and asked if my parents were around so we could have a family meeting. I said, my mom is, and texted her to come back immediately.

Dr. Mohabir said that my prognosis is not good. People who

have been on IVs for THIS long, who are incapable of being off antibiotics, don't turn around. The bacteria just don't let up at any point. He said there probably won't be a time in the future when I'll be able to stay healthy without antibiotics; he said that the antibiotics are propping my lung function up and keeping me alive. Without the antibiotics, he said, I wouldn't live for another year.

He said some people get to the point that they can't do it anymore. They go off the antibiotics, their lung function plummets, and then they get listed for transplant. But with me, it's not so easy—no center wants to transplant me. He said he's talked about me to many centers who said no. They are not excited about me as a *candidate,* were the words he used. But he thinks Duke, Toronto, and Pittsburgh are three that could still be options. He said he was going to see if they'd be willing to talk with me. According to Dr. Mohabir, the problem is that I'm in cepacia syndrome. A slow version of it. He said that when he tells the centers that I have *cepacia* and I'm in syndrome, they immediately assume I'll just die on the table. Because that's what happens when you try to transplant with cepacia syndrome. The outcomes are just not good.

Obviously, I don't want to push to get on a transplant list and expedite that process just to get a surgery I don't feel confident I'll survive. I want to prolong my life as long as possible. But at the same time, I feel like as I'm working so hard to stay alive, I need to have some kind of backup plan—I need to know that when the IVs eventually stop holding me steady and my lung function plummets, there will be a center that will list me. At that point, I'll pack my bags and be on the first plane. I don't want that to happen anytime soon, but I want to know whether it's even a possibility for my future. I want to know if there's a center that will take me, and ideally, which one.

He said that I should not expect to be off IVs for any significant length of time, and that I should not get my hopes up about
transplant. He said they are still tweaking and changing the regimen to fight each exacerbation as it comes, but, looking at things
on a macro scale, and based on my last year and what he knows
from his experience treating others with *cepacia,* he believes that
my *cepacia* is now a superbug—and it is not going to get better.
The infection is going to take over. The antibiotics are slowing
that process down. I will have to be on them as long as I can stand
it, as long as they keep working, or as long as it's safe to (e.g., if I
start to have kidney failure, we might need to reevaluate).

As he was saying this, it seemed like he thought there was a
chance I might give up—that I might say, essentially, I can't do
this anymore. I can't be on these IVs for weeks, months, maybe
years more. He said other patients have just "given up" and gone
home on hospice. And he acknowledged my quality of life has
been shot to hell, even though my lung function is 45 percent.

Now I feel like I've sort of been living in a delusion. When I
started my period of sickness one year ago, I kept thinking, for the
first few rounds of IVs, that I would get better and bounce back
and get back to life. In L.A., I began to lose hope as the months
wore on and I got worse and worse, losing more and more
strength, more and more weight, and more and more reason to
live. Everything was slipping away. I was completely depressed. I
was anxious all the time and had no faith. No faith in my body,
no faith in the doctors' ability to fix me, no faith that my life
would go back to the way it was.

But when I moved to S.F., even though I was on long-term
IVs, it was like this dormant part of me was awakened again by the
simple fact of being around friends. It was like drinking Red Bulls
and taking happy pills. I felt like myself again, even though I
wasn't surfing, even though I wasn't playing volleyball, even

though I was on IVs, even though I was away from the beach. I reconnected with my motivated, intellectual side. I got down to business, I finished Susan's book and did other writing. And I worked out. Set goals. Made plans. Explored the city and deepened my relationships with people from my college community, people I had drifted from when I lived in L.A. It was a beautiful high, a beautiful first couple of months here.

So, yes, I was living in a delusion. I thought that after a certain amount of time on IVs, I would just miraculously not need them anymore and be better. In reality, when I went off IVs, I got sick two weeks later and was back on IVs four weeks later. I did not get much time at all, and since I've gone back on them, I've been hospitalized three times. It's all becoming a blur, and that's the worst fucking part.

Anyway. Back to Mohabir's talk. He said it was time to start living my life.

This was one of the most emotional talks I've had in my entire life. My mom was bawling her eyes out. I was trying to be strong for her, and trying to hold it together, but I was crying, too.

At the very beginning, back when I was young, I used to cough up blood on the pool deck, but I was naive and excited and happy and growing and changing and trying. Now my heart breaks for that little girl because she thought she had a long future, and my current reality is telling me that I don't.

And my heart breaks for my mom and dad. They just want to keep me alive and they will do whatever they can to make that happen. I try to do my part, and I think I do my best. But I also have to live my life. And that's the part Dr. Mohabir was emphasizing. I think he was trying to explain that I might not have that much time. Because how long can one really be on these IVs? A few years, sure, maybe, that would be a long time for IVs, but a few years is not a long time to live. It's crazy to think that when

I'm around twenty-six, when my friends are moving in with their boyfriends or getting married or starting business school or having kids or getting promoted or doing whatever the hell they're doing, I could be packing up to move to North Carolina, Toronto, Pittsburgh, or Cleveland. That is such a mind-fuck. Picturing my mom in snow boots would almost be enough to make me laugh, if I weren't crying. And would my dad come? What about Micah?

When Dr. Mohabir was talking, he kept circling back to the idea of doing what makes me happy. And I kept thinking about people. Not places I want to go or bucket list things I want to do. It was about the people I love, getting enough time with them. Not feeling like I'm leaving them behind. Or being left behind myself, while their lives all move on. That's the problem with death. For everyone else, it's an event, it's sad and shitty and grief-inducing, but then life goes on. For the deceased, that's it, that's the end.

I'm afraid of what's to come. In some ways, I feel like nothing will change. When I leave here, I'll—hopefully—be feeling a little better. I'll be on a home IV regimen. Ideally, we'll go on a vacation to Hawaii. Whether or not we choose to take the risk and go to Hawaii, afterward, I'll come back and still be on IVs. And that could go on indefinitely. Maybe I won't be hospitalized again for months; maybe it'll just be weeks. Who knows? Nobody knows how fast this thing will progress. I think we're all just relieved that my high fevers have stopped and that, so far, there's no growth in my blood cultures. Which means that at this particular time, the antibiotics are still helping—all seven of them. It's not feasible to go home on all of them, so we'll have to figure out a way to send me home with IVs I can manage.

Dr. Chhatwani rounded the next day and told me that I need to accept more help than I've had until now. For example, I might need a home health nurse who comes and does IVs. Or have someone else who comes to help even if they don't do the IVs. Or have family live in the area to help me.

Having family stay with me aligns with my goal of having Kona up here (that was one of the things I realized when I started thinking about my time being limited. I want my dog in my life. Literally all I wanted to do when I was talking to Dr. M was to cry into Kona's fur).

It was an extremely dire prognosis. But it wasn't new information. Dr. M was just flicking on the lights so we could see what everyone else already had seen—that *cepacia* has taken over, and it's time to figure out a transplant option.

I realize I want to write my story.

The thing that I haven't even processed yet, and I'm tearing up thinking about it now, is that I won't have a family. I really want to have a family. I want to get married and have kids (or adopt—since I've always known I wouldn't be able to carry my own kids). I have multiple Word documents filled with names for future children. I've always loved names. And family. And the idea of having my own kids. I think it's because I'm twenty-three that this feels like an especially hard thing to let go of. It's not something I ever foresaw having to sacrifice, for some reason. Which goes to show that some part of me has always been living with the delusion that I'd live a long and healthy life.

I'm scared. And I think I'm falling in love with Jack. And I don't know if that's just because of the shit storm I'm going through, and the fact that he happens to be there, or if it's him, but I think it's happening. It almost feels weird that we don't say the words "I love you," because our dynamic is so loving. I have to stop myself from saying "love you" whenever I say goodbye or good night. I don't know if he feels the same way, but I know he has been deeply affected by the events of this week.

The night he found out I might only have a year left, he cried so hard. I never thought I would see him cry like that, and I was so surprised, because when my mom and I were first explaining things to him, he was sort of staring off into a corner, seeming very distant and apathetic. In the middle of this my dad arrived (my mom had said it was urgent he come). And then as soon as my parents left the room he started crying, and I realized that he had just been trying not to cry. But once he did start crying, he completely broke down.

That's a whole long story, though, the story of that night. The short version is: he was devastated, he was crying, he said he didn't know how to be strong for me. I told him that he didn't need to be strong by not crying, he was doing exactly what he should be doing as a boyfriend by showing up and calling. I told him he's doing all the right things, and it absolutely does not bother me for him to show emotion and cry around me. In fact, it was touching to me, because it showed me how deeply he cares.

I truly did not know how he was going to react to this information. He said he didn't know if he could ever just be light-hearted around me again, if he could just go on vacation and have fun without just being sad all the time. And I kind of made the comparison that I don't know if he's leaving in the fall, and so it's similar in that I, too, don't know what the future holds, and I, too, am scared, but that doesn't mean we should back away from it.

We talked for a long time. He cried, we hugged, we laughed. The crazy thing is that I had cried all that day, and have cried so many times since that day, but I did not cry one time that night. It was like my body was empty of tears. By the time he left, he said he was feeling much better, much more optimistic. He said he wasn't scared anymore and whatever happened, we would tackle it together. It was so incredibly sweet.

My mom wrote on Facebook so we wouldn't have to repeat the story over and over:

> There's no way to sugarcoat this message. Mallory Smith's long-term prognosis is not good. She has been fighting the worst possible bacteria for a very long time and it seems the antibiotic options that she's been on have run their course. The doctors are making tweaks but don't think it's likely that things will turn around.
>
> It's clear that most people don't understand the severity of the situation because Mallory looks so good and does so much. We felt it was time to let our beloved family and friends know how difficult things are for her.
>
> The doctors don't think Mallory's health can be sustained without IVs so the plan is to keep her on them indefinitely. Hopefully that will allow her to have some quality of life. Mallory wants to do as much as possible for as long as possible.
>
> The Stanford team is talking to transplant centers around the country to try to find one that will consider Mallory as a candidate. But they are not optimistic because of the bacteria she cultures. We live in hope.
>
> She has finally agreed to write her story.

Now it's 12:30 and I should sleep. I'm sure I left out much of what happened this week. There's just no way to retain all of this. And I'm pissed that I've had to take so much Ativan because it's messing with my memory.

8/4/16—Mark Smith

*After Stanford rejected Mallory as a candidate for transplant, citing the
risk caused by her* B. cepacia *infection, I started desperately looking for
ways to mitigate that risk. My research led me to an article called "Ef-
ficacy of bacteriophage therapy in a model of* Burkholderia cenocepacia *pulmonary infection" in the* Journal of Infectious Diseases *by
John J. LiPuma, M.D., a professor of pediatrics at the University of
Michigan and the director of the Burkholderia cepacia Research Labora-
tory and Repository.*

*Bacteriophages (phages) are naturally occurring viruses that have
evolved to attack bacteria. Unlike chemical antibiotics, they are target-
specific: each variety of phage attacks only one species of bacteria, sometimes only one particular strain. The idea behind phage therapy is to find
several phages active against a particular strain of bacteria, grow them in a
culture of those bacteria, purify them, and then administer them to a patient to eradicate the bacterial infection.*

*Diane and I had directed funds from our annual fundraiser to
Dr. LiPuma's lab for many years, so I reached out to him by email.
Dr. LiPuma had not continued the line of investigation outlined in his
article. He referred me to Jonathan Dennis, Ph.D., of the University of
Alberta, who was apparently continuing to investigate phage therapy.*

*According to Dr. Dennis, phages, or combinations of phages, exist
that can kill any particular strain of bacteria. His lab had used phages to
eradicate* B. cepacia *infection from the lungs of cystic fibrosis knockout
mice. But he had not been able to try it on humans. He had worked with
clinicians from around the world, including Australia, Germany, and the
United States. Phage therapy looked feasible several times, but each time,
even with end-of-life candidate trials, liability issues did not allow the application to proceed.*

*Dr. Dennis wrote, "Everyone is waiting for clinical trials to be con-
ducted that, if successful, will permit the FDA to approve phage therapy,*

at least in some cases. . . . Based upon the science, phage therapy should be effective. Legally, I do not know how to go about this."

Funding for phage therapy was just not available. Pharmaceutical companies were not interested, apparently because the end product would not be a patentable chemical.

I suggested to Diane and Mallory that we fund Dr. Dennis's research into phage therapy. They declined, thinking it was a long shot that would not be clinically available in time to help Mallory.

I discontinued my research into phage therapy.

8/5/16

Feeling a little emotionally numb. It's now Friday so I've been here in Stanford Hospital for a week and four days. I'm supposed to be getting out on Monday.

Today I got calls from Cleveland Clinic and University of Pittsburgh Medical Center (UPMC), from their transplant programs, to verify some information. It was shitty false hope from Cleveland because the medical director of their transplant program had already told my mom by email that they have a blanket policy against transplanting *cenocepacia* patients, and they already told Chhatwani that they wouldn't consider me. But UPMC!!!!! I'm still hopeful.

But what do you call it when the best-case scenario, the thing you're hoping for, is almost as terrifying as death itself? This week, time and again, I've thought about the fact that the road will only get harder from here. And I don't know if I should try to forget that, to distract myself from that, or if I should really reflect on it so that I can be grateful for the health that I do have now. Because on the one hand, understanding how hard things will be in the future does make me realize how lucky I still am. But on the other hand, I am scared shitless about what the future will bring, for how much I will suffer, and for how much my family will suffer.

The thing I keep thinking about, the image I keep coming back to, is a reservoir. My family's love for me and their ability to help me is this reservoir that seems endlessly deep. It always seems like it will never run out. But as things get harder and as I deplete their resources (their love, their time, their money, their concern), I know we will get to a point where we *have* to worry about running out. I don't know if we will run out of money—my parents are literally buying the apartment beneath mine in a city that I don't even know how much longer I'll live in just to be there for me—or if I will just suck them dry, until the only thing they're living for is me and they have nothing left. I already feel like I've taken so much away from them and now my mom has to uproot herself to move up here and live with me.

That's one issue.

Another issue is that I don't know what to do about my vacation—whether to go to Hawaii or not. Whether to plan a different trip.

I feel awful that I've burdened Jack with so much worry about me when he's in his second-to-last quarter at Stanford and he's worked his entire life to get here and now he's tanking his GPA. I just can't imagine the stress that he's feeling. But I also can't be worried too much about his stress because I have to worry about my own stress and, fundamentally, the one who's going through this is me. I am not minimizing what he's going through. He has to be absolutely torn about how to handle this.

He says he's on the verge of tears all the time and yet he has to go to office hours, attend class, work in his lab, etc. He has to put on a brave face in front of my friends and family and his own friends. I guess he's just picturing the worst possible scenarios in his mind and that's what's so hard for him—he says he's freaking out all the time. He's worried he'll just be walking to class and get a call that something catastrophic has happened to me. It's beauti-

ful that he cares enough to be so distraught over what's going on
with me.

But when he disappeared for a few days it was hard for me to
not know if he was coming, or if I was going to hear from him. If
he was having doubts, I would rather have known. I would understand. Completely. He only has one quarter left at Stanford
after this, and if he wants to focus on school and friends, I would
understand. Especially since he's likely going to move away anyway. I don't think he wants out because he hasn't said anything
like that. I am trying to give him space but then I wonder, why?
And where do we stand as a couple?

I really care about him a lot. I almost said "I love you" the other
night, but then I didn't, because I didn't want to complicate things
even further. Now I'm especially happy that I didn't say that, given
that he's been having an awful time adjusting to what's going on
with me, and that I don't know if he wants to stay together.

That brings me back to vacation. Perhaps I should make a
decision about Hawaii independent of his scheduling constraints.
If I do end up being able to go to Hawaii but not at a time that
works for him, it will still be nice; what I want is to surf, to be in
the water, etc. If I can't go with Jack, so be it. It would've been
fun, especially if Michelle and Matt could go as planned. But after
talking to Caleigh, who doesn't think it's a good idea for me to
go, I'm second-guessing the idea of going in two weeks. It might
be fine to just go to Malibu, go for some nice drives, stay in a nice
house, and do some hikes.

I feel like I've given up in the fight a bit. . . . I feel so unmo-
tivated to get back to my life, to get back to work. I feel a lack of
optimism that I will ever be able to do the things I love. If I can't
be the person I was, I don't know who to become. I don't know
how to prioritize my health without being just a sick person. I

don't know how to explain this situation to my friends, how to talk about my prognosis, how to conceive of how much time I have left, and how to prioritize what I do with that time.

8/8/16

Got discharged from the hospital today. But I don't feel as happy as I think I should. I vaguely remember, in my recent hospitalizations, feeling really excited to get back to S.F. and my apartment. But now I don't feel excited.

It scares me how dependent I am on so many medications. I feel extremely dysphoric, just generally dissatisfied with life. And I can see logically from the outside that I have no reason to feel that way. Well, I do have some reason. I did just get news that my prognosis is horrible, and every few days I get more rejections from transplant centers. So yes, I have reasons to feel sad. But usually I can compartmentalize and still find happiness in the present moment. Today I just felt like I would never be happy again. Except when I was with Jack—I felt happy when he came over. So even if our relationship ends after this fall, I think it's worth it to be with him until then because he brings me happiness.

Later that day, Julia and Liane came over and we hung out with Tamara, who was still visiting. It was so great to have friends over! We went back out to a table by the fountain in front of the hospital. Caleigh and her mom, Lizeth, came outside at the same time, so we all chatted. It broke my heart to see Caleigh. She weighs sixty-seven pounds now and she can't eat a thing because she's nauseous and vomiting. It's just heartbreaking how much she suffers. She's so skinny, she's super fragile, but that girl just doesn't break. I wonder often how she keeps her spirits up. I think it might be her family. They seem to bring her a lot of joy.

She told me that when she was waiting for transplant but

thought she might not survive long enough to get one, she started marking off bucket list items. That made me want to create a bucket list. I've been living so safely that I feel like I don't even have an adventurous spirit anymore. Caleigh found a hot air balloon company that let her bring oxygen up in the air, somewhere near Napa. That blew my mind. I'm so much healthier now than she was when she did that, and she had more spirit than I do. It was like a kick in the ass to do things.

But at the same time, I feel like I want to protect myself, because if I can't get a transplant, then I have to keep myself stable or I'll die. Everything feels very hopeless right now and I'm trying to find a way to convince my brain to feel hope. But I can't when that doesn't seem logical.

8/10/16

August is a big birthday month in the Smith family. My mom's birthday is today, my dad's sixtieth is Friday, and Micah's twenty-sixth is in twelve days.

I am limited in what I can do, but not in what I can say. The biggest challenge I've faced in the past year has not been keeping myself healthy—it has been trying to adequately express my gratitude to my family for the insane, over-the-top, unbelievable sacrifices they've made to further my well-being. For nearly twenty-four years, their needs have been secondary to my own.

To say they are the best parents I could ever ask for sounds trite. To say I am grateful is an understatement. A Facebook post can't do them justice. It feels absurd to try to thank them with words— I wish I could plan a six-month vacation for them, to thank them for bending over backward every single day to keep me alive.

It's the beginning of a new chapter for all of us. I am grateful to my mom, to my dad, and to Micah, for never making me feel guilty about all that they've had to give up. They are amazing.

8/24/16

I look around and see blue. Royal blue water, turquoise farther in the distance. Blue cloudless sky. Even the boat is blue.

My back bakes in the sun and my right foot sizzles. My right arm wraps tightly around Jack—after a year away from the ocean, getting tossed off a fast-moving boat in water hundreds of feet deep would be traumatic.

My breath quickens as the wind and swell pick up. I remind myself to breathe deeply and slowly, knowing that anxiety-induced breathlessness is the one kind I can control. As I maintain my death grip on the rope and focus on my long inhale-exhales, it hits me all at once—I'm in Hawaii. In the middle of the ocean. My favorite place, and my other favorite place. I'm not in a hospital. I'm with Jack, Michelle, Matt, Ari, and Justin. Even Micah is here! It's sunny, it's beautiful. I can breathe. I'm not wearing oxygen. No one on the boat that didn't know me would think there was anything wrong with me, other than a cough. I'm happy, happier than I can remember being in a long time.

We continue on toward Molokini and I smile and smile. I wonder again if this is the last time I'll ever come to Hawaii, and then I banish that thought and look down at the water, noticing the way the boat cuts through it so forcefully yet so elegantly. It's a beautiful Wednesday.

I keep wondering: Can this be real life? I think, maybe my life can be like this again. Maybe I can walk on the beach and do long open-water swims and start surfing again. Maybe I can help with the dishes and not freak out over a bad night of sleep. Already, in just six days, showering normally has stopped feeling remarkable; maybe, just maybe, I'll stay off IVs long enough that submerging underwater will stop feeling like a long-lost vestige from my past.

I'm just so happy to be here. Even though I can't dive as deep as I could when I was a kid. Even though I can't surf at all, when just a year ago I was charging. I lugged my oxygen concentrator to the beach (or rather, Jack lugged it). Things are different now, we know that. But in some ways, everything is the same—the same peace descends each time I jump in the water, the same euphoria when a sea turtle or a reef shark swims below me. The same simple pleasure comes from eating big dinners with family and friends, from sitting on our patio with wine and cheese.

8/25/16

I sit on the lanai of our condo in ninety-degree weather in a long-sleeve shirt, sweatshirt, yoga pants, and a second layer of sweatpants on top. My body won't stop shivering, so I'm searching for the warmest place I can find. Jack comes out onto the patio to get the grill ready to cook leg of lamb. I know I'll have to leave the patio when the grill gets smoky, and I wonder where I can go to avoid freezing. The bedroom is out of the question—the fan and A/C keep it a frigid sixty-eight degrees. My parents' bedroom is even colder.

Finally, I drag myself up off the outdoor sofa, the bag with my oxygen concentrator draped over me cross-body style, pulling my shoulders forward. Into the bathroom I go, where I pull out the blow-dryer and start blow-drying my already-dry hair, face, neck, chest, back, legs. Anxiety begins to set in; it's completely illogical to feel hypothermic in ninety-degree heat. But when does my body ever act in a way that's logical? It's illogical to get sick while on three oral antibiotics, two inhaled antibiotics, and thirty-five other medications. Since my life never feels logical, blow-drying my entire body in a bathroom in Hawaii doesn't even feel that crazy.

But a case of severe chills, for me, is ominous. When I eventually take my temperature, I have a fever of 103.3. My stomach drops.

. . .

It's a couple of hours after my fever spiked above 103, and I'm in the emergency room at Maui Memorial Medical Center. Before the trip, we'd looked up the hospital on the island to find out if it had an ICU, an interventional radiology team, and experienced pulmonologists. I didn't think I would end up needing their services; mostly, the research was meant to convince my Stanford medical team that I'd done my homework and had fully thought through my decision to take the trip.

The IV alarm blares like a siren, a foot away from my head. After five minutes of sleep, the IV antibiotic has finished, and the pump won't let me forget it. I press the call button for the nurse to come shut off the alarm so I can catch a few minutes of sleep before going to my next test. No one comes, so I fiddle with some buttons on the pump, familiar enough with how they work by now to silence it temporarily.

After a long night in the emergency room, I get admitted to the step-down ICU at Maui Memorial. Dr. Mohabir calls to check in on me at 4:00 a.m. Hawaii time, but I'm finally asleep, so he leaves a voicemail.

Dr. M tells my mom that he wants me out of the hospital in twenty-four hours. He wants me to enjoy the rest of my vacation, just with home IV antibiotics. That means no time in the water, but I'm learning that there's more to life than plan A. The particulars of plan B—R&R, good meals, reclining in the shade with a good book—sound pretty damn good right about now. Better than staying in a hospital bed for another few weeks, getting weaker, waiting for the drugs to suppress this infection.

I've quoted this saying from a fellow CF-er before, but it just hits so close to home: Reality always finds us. Being in the hospital and on IVs is my reality, as much as I would love to play hide-and-seek, staying healthy and hidden on an island forever.

Before reality found me, I got to do things that bring me unadulterated joy for six straight days. The infection caught up to me, but I have two words for it: game on!

8/31/16

When I got out of the hospital we went back to the condo. Things were okay for a few days but I started to deteriorate on Saturday and got even worse on Sunday.

That night we were trying to decide what to do. We were supposed to stay until Thursday but there was news that a hurricane was coming. I started to panic about getting stuck on the island. Jack was great. He listened to me sob. It was the anniversary of Kari's death and that also rattled me. It was all crashing down on me. The future felt too hard. Jack didn't know what to say, how could he? But he listened, and he was present. And he made me feel safe. He had to get back to school and I didn't want to stay on without him.

My mom jumped through lots of hoops to change all of our tickets to get us off the island (clearly others had the same idea to cut their trip short). She was ultimately able to make the arrangements and we flew the next day.

The crazy thing was that as we were rushing to pack and get to the airport, UPMC called to say I was approved for the evaluation. I was in the middle of treatment, everyone else was scrambling to pack up, so I handed the phone to my mom, who tried to stay calm as she attempted to capture important details about the weeklong process. She was clearly struggling to stay focused as she was processing her overwhelming joy. None of us could believe this was really happening.

The call took a long time. We were late getting to the airport and carrying so much medical gear. The hurricane was imminent, and that, combined with my high fever, made for an intense travel day. I was so relieved when we touched down, even though Hawaii had been absolutely incredible.

For a few days, being in Maui and seeing all that I could do made that prognosis I had received from Stanford seem ridiculous. How I felt the first few days of the trip gave me hope that I could reclaim my old life again, my old identity. That hope felt good. Even now that I'm back in Stanford Hospital, battling the same old infection, running through the same old tiresome drill, I feel a little more hopeful.

Some might think it was irresponsible to take an IV holiday so soon after the doctors said I couldn't survive off IVs. But life is a balancing act—as patients, we have to keep our bodies healthy, yes, but also our minds. We have to know that there's life out there to be lived, however sick we get. Whatever it takes to remind us of that is worth it, in my eyes. Calculated risk-taking is the name of the game for me now, rather than cautious sheltering.

I do know now with 100 percent certainty that I made the right choice to go. And the right choice to come back, as it's pointless to stick to a vacation plan if you're so sick that being away from your doctor is terrifying. Both were such huge decisions, it was hard to know what to do. Going was enormous, canceling our last few days in Hawaii was enormous, deciding to land and head straight to the ER without unpacking or getting resettled was enormous, but my gut was telling me that I needed to be back in my second home. I needed to be evaluated.

9/1/16

Two big developments with Jack!

First, his dad wants to meet me!!! Jack sent this text: *"My dad *wants to meet you. That's super rare. He even choked up on the phone when he told me how proud he was that I have been able to find a way to support you even though you've been going through so much. You're the real champ in my eyes, but he can tell you've made me a better person. I know your parents thank me all the time for the things I do for you, but I just want to make it clear that there is an equal amount of thanks to you for the things you do for me. In short, thanks for continuing to be awesome, everyone can see it, not just me."*

Second, he came to the hospital today (it's now Thursday, I came in to the ER on Tuesday) and we hung out all afternoon and he said he loves me for the first time! He said, "I care about you so much," and I said, "So do I." And then he said, "I love you, Mallory," and I said I loved him back!

It was a beautiful moment. I'd been in severe pain all day with this pleuritic chest pain and really frustrated by the lack of coordination/responsiveness in my pain management. I'd also been feeling dejected about being back here again. But then Jack came and it perked me up, and we went on a walk by the fountain, and he said he loved me!!!!!!!!

Where I am with work/professional/creative endeavors:

I'm editing David's book. Want to stay on top of that and work faster but also do a very, very good job.

I need to start thinking about what I want to do for my own book. So many people have reached out to offer to get me an agent or have it read by a publisher! I need to make something of this and capitalize on the fact that I'm starting down this whole transplant road and that this is the time in my life where shit gets complicated and interesting.

My updates are scatterbrained because I'm on drugs (prescribed ones, of course).

9/10/16

I'm in L.A. now, came to visit my grandma, who was diagnosed with end-stage ovarian cancer. It's just so sad. She and my grandpa were so much a part of my growing up.

I'm feeling sad about so many things but also worried about transplant. I hope Pittsburgh has some redeeming qualities, I really do. Something to make me think that living there for a few years, potentially even dying there, wouldn't be the worst thing in the world. I have to be able to find joy there, otherwise what's the point?

Today, I woke up before 10:00 a.m. (I've been waking up at like noon every day, so 10:00 a.m. is an achievement). I ate a normal breakfast (oatmeal, fruit, and coffee) and felt fine afterward, did treatment and worked on David's book (reedited chapter 3). I felt focused, then went to work out at Grandma's gym. (Fifteen minutes on the elliptical, thank God for supplemental oxygen, then weights, then foam rolled.) After that, I went upstairs and talked to Grandpa for a long time and visited with Grandma. Hanging out with Grandpa was really nice. I sat there with him and ate a frozen peach and listened to his stories of the old days.

Going into Grandma's room I started to get emotional. She said that now was the time she was supposed to tell everyone the last things she wanted to say to them, so she was going to tell me something. "Mallory, ever since you were a little girl, I've thought you were extraordinary," she said. "But as you've grown up, you get more extraordinary every day. I'm so proud to be your grandma, and I claim no credit for how amazing you've turned out. But I love you so much and I'm lucky to be your grandma." I started crying, because how could I not? Her diagnosis is so devastating.

Being with them was very emotional and after I left, I didn't feel like seeing anybody so I walked home (which was almost a mile, more than I've walked in a very long time). While I walked

I listened to music and cried more. I was thinking about Grandma being sick, but also about what will happen to Grandpa when she dies, and what on earth he would do if we all had to move to the East Coast for me to get a transplant.

I'm also not ready to say goodbye to my life yet—my friends and my social life, Maria, Micah, Kona, Grandma and Grandpa, Northern California crisp air and trees and routines, Southern California beach days and lazy afternoons. All the little things that make up the familiar. I'm not ready to transform my life yet.

I was also thinking about how my mom doesn't deserve to have a parent die and a daughter die close together in time, so I need to live a long time for her because she deserves better than all this sadness. I worry about how my dad would survive losing me. I don't know if my parents' marriage could survive that much sadness, and I think if I were to die, my main wish would be for them to lean into each other to get through it rather than pull away from each other. I would hope that if anything ever happened to me, it would bring my family closer together, not fracture them apart.

9/11/16

I've been thinking about the concept of "mind over matter" a lot lately as I try to reframe the way I view my own future. I'm working very hard to see beauty in a life that will look quite different from the one I wanted and expected. I'm trying to see adventure in the possibility of moving to Pittsburgh or Toronto even though I hate the cold, I'm not much of an urbanite, and I live for the ocean. I'm trying to see hope when the data tells me that people with my bacterial infection usually die on the operating table or within a year post-transplant. I'm trying not to think about how few years I might have left and instead focus on how much life I've already lived in the twenty-four-ish years I've been alive. I'm trying to focus my attention on the incredible, fleeting moments of joy—like sprawling on a couch with five of my close friends, laughing so hard I can barely breathe—rather than on the periods of uncertainty, fear, and anxiety. Those joyous moments are the ones I want to convert to long-term memory; the other ones I could do to let go of. Ruminating won't help one bit.

"Mind over matter" is a powerful tool to press the reset button, to change the narrative of a life, to see the sparkle of a gemstone in a mound of rubble. But it only works when we see our reality for what it really is, and then pick and choose which pieces of that reality to emphasize. It's not about deluding ourselves by saying a life-threatening genetic disorder is not a disease; such rhetoric doesn't help us, the disabled—it only helps those who are uncomfortable witnessing our health challenges.

In September, I traveled to L.A. to see family and friends. In October, I will travel to Pittsburgh for a transplant evaluation and then celebrate my birthday. In November, I will go to L.A. again for my annual CF fundraiser (An Evening in Mallory's Garden) and Thanksgiving.

Throughout these months, I will continue working (part-time, from home). I will continue writing. I will continue to despise red Jell-O. I will hopefully stay out of the hospital for a while (no promises there), but I will continue on IVs. I will get myself back into the gym, into the yoga studio, or onto the streets to walk. I will probably not drink any apple cider vinegar, because it's gross and it burns my throat. I will be utterly compliant with my treatments and medications. I will hope for the best and prepare for the worst.

And, mostly, I will understand that I'm fighting a motherfucker of a disease, that it's extremely hard work, and that I'm doing the best I can.

10/2/16

Last Thursday at midnight, after twelve hours of travel with six medical bags and an oxygen tank, my mom and I touched down in Pittsburgh International Airport. It was supposed to be the start of our *Thelma and Louise* adventure. In fact, it was the day from hell.

Packing up all the mechanical and chemical paraphernalia that keep me alive was tough. We had to bring my vest machine, compressor, nebulizers, oxygen tank and its accessories, forty-plus pounds of IV medications, twenty-two different kinds of pills, and inhaled medications. With my foggy mind, limited energy, shortness of breath, low oxygen, and midday vomiting, it was a grueling effort. But we got it done, and Thursday morning we packed up the car to go to the airport.

People often ask why *B. cepacia* is contraindicated for transplant. The reasons are multifaceted:

1. Transplant centers need to keep their one-year survival rates above a certain percentage (80 or 90 percent) in order to stay in business: if they fall below national standards, their program risks being shut down. Transplant is a huge moneymaker for hospitals, so staying in business is a top priority. Taking on high-risk cases such as patients with *cenocepacia* can compromise outcomes.
2. Lungs are a scarce commodity. There are not enough organ donors in the United States to supply lungs to all the people waiting. Many patients die on the list. Ethically speaking, I think it's hard to give lungs to someone who doesn't have a good chance of making it when they could go to a less risky patient with a higher chance of survival.
3. Doctors are obligated under the Hippocratic Oath to do no harm. If the data shows that most patients with *B. cepacia* either die on the table or within a year after transplant, some feel it is

more harmful to try the risky procedure than not to—even if not trying means the patient will die.

4. The timing of a transplant is also complicated. There is a small window in which patients are eligible for transplant; they have to be so sick that they can't live long without new lungs, but healthy enough to survive the operation. A patient can become too sick for transplant very abruptly, losing eligibility. Right now, given that a transplant for me would require a cross-country move, I'm in the window where I need to start the process, need to complete the full evaluation. If my health all of a sudden plummeted, I couldn't just go to the closest ICU and get listed for transplant there, so I need to plan ahead.

5. The timing of a transplant involving *B. cepacia* carries an additional layer of complication since *cepacia* and *cenocepacia* can cause "cepacia syndrome" at any time. Cepacia syndrome is a fatal, necrotizing pneumonia that can kill within days or weeks.

The timing of transplant and the fact that it can only be done in Pittsburgh are important parts of the story I'm about to tell, a classic story of the big corporation screwing the little guy, of the large-scale forces at work in healthcare jeopardizing a patient's life. For me, the story is new, but countless others have already lived this story. And, spoiler alert: it does not always have a happy ending.

When we first got the call from Pittsburgh's intake coordinator, she brought up the financial burden of transplant. The coordinator warned us that with our insurance, Blue Cross, we would undoubtedly face problems getting coverage for the evaluation (not to mention the transplant), since UPMC is not an in-network provider for them. They told us to start pushing Blue Cross immediately. It was about five weeks before the evaluation.

My mom started the process. Predictably, Blue Cross wrote us a letter explaining that they would not provide coverage for an evaluation at UPMC because it was not an in-network hospital. They recommended that I seek care at Minnesota. Obviously, they failed to understand that I have zero choice when it comes to where I get my transplant and that Minnesota had already rejected my case. Dozens of phone calls ensued as my mom struggled to get past the lowest person on the totem pole, a woman who was tasked with delivering us the bad news and who had no power to change anything. She was the wall Blue Cross put up; unfailingly polite, she said no, no, no.

Four times the coordinator would call and tell my mom that we needed to consider a particular center. Each time my mom would say they won't take Mallory. Blue Cross would then say give us five days to check. Then they would call back, say my mom was right but that we had to try another Blue Cross–approved center. This obvious stall tactic set us back weeks.

Finally, somehow, my mom got a verbal agreement from Blue Cross to issue the paperwork to provide a ninety-day authorization for me to see the transplant team at UPMC. They were not covering transplant, just the evaluation, but they confirmed that this was indeed an authorization.

When they sent the paperwork, they wrote in the name of the wrong hospital (there are many hospitals in Pittsburgh). We asked them to correct it and to send the paperwork back again, and they said they would. Again, when the paperwork came in, the name was wrong—the hospital they wrote in is not even tangentially associated with UPMC cardiothoracic transplant.

At this point, our suspicions were confirmed that Blue Cross's bureaucratic obstacles were intentional stall tactics. Days and weeks were passing, and the date of my cross-country trip was getting closer and closer. We reckoned that the low woman on the totem pole was being instructed to do whatever she needed to do to prevent me from getting evaluated at Pittsburgh.

All the while, I was in L.A. because of my grandma's end-stage cancer diagnosis. I was sick and did not have the energy to keep track of this ongoing battle myself. Ever since I graduated high school, I've been fiercely independent when it comes to my medical care, handling all interactions with doctors, hospitals, co-ordinators, and pharmacies. But when it came to insurance, I just couldn't do it. While I rested in bed, I heard my mom screaming on the phone in her office. She spent hours and hours during those few weeks fighting Blue Cross, precious hours she could have spent taking care of her own mom and dad.

Blue Cross called back and said they had done the paperwork right, and they said (over the phone) that I was approved. I was good to go. They said they would send the paperwork directly to UPMC. Everything was set, as far as we knew; our appointments were scheduled, my transplant binder came in the mail, our flights were booked, hotel rooms reserved. We had won this first battle— or so we thought.

But then, in the car ride to the airport for the flight to Pittsburgh, we were blindsided by a bait and switch so egregious it seems criminal. A woman who does insurance verification for UPMC called. She said that I had no insurance approval on file at UPMC whatsoever, and thus, that she would have to cancel all of my appointments for the upcoming week. When I told her that she was wrong, that I had already gotten Blue Cross's approval for the evaluation, she got angry and hung up on me.

My fatigue at that point was bone crushing, as if my limbs were lead and my head was filled with bricks. My mom took over, and her first call was to the lung transplant coordinator at UPMC who had been helping us. What is going on??? This was the essence of her side of the conversation: We started this process over a month ago. How can they promise us approval, and then withdraw that approval when we're already on the way to the

airport?? According to the coordinator, Blue Cross never officially
sent in the authorization. They lied to us, pretended that it was
taken care of when it wasn't, and waited until the very last minute
to tell us that we couldn't ultimately get coverage, when it could
have very well been too late to fix. My mom told UPMC that we
were coming, insurance or no insurance.

Hell hath no fury like a mom who thinks someone is getting
in the way of her daughter's transplant evaluation.

As I sat on the first leg of the flight, headed to Charlotte,
North Carolina, I stewed. I could not live with the idea that I
could potentially be going through such a grueling day of travel
to end up in Pittsburgh with NO appointments. Beyond the implications for my own health, it made me wonder what happens
to the patients who don't have parents who are willing and able to
draft 800-word emails, to scream at people on the phone, to
threaten legal action (my dad) or a publicist's wrath (my mom)?
While in many ways I'm in a position of complete powerlessness
at the hands of a company that cares more about their bottom line
than about whether I survive (in fact, one that would probably
rather I die, because it would be cheaper), I still have an advantage
that many patients aren't lucky enough to possess: two dedicated,
tenacious, educated parents with the resources to fight the system.

It occurred to me in a heartbreaking moment that the patients who don't have that are the patients who die as a result of
bureaucratic bullshit. It's so absurd it makes me shake with rage.
When you're in need of a lung transplant, and the people on the
other end of the line are intentionally trying to block you from
getting lifesaving care, and you're weary and you don't have parents to fight your battles, you die.

Studies show that cancer patients with bad insurance die at
higher rates than their counterparts with better coverage. This sad
reality is true of CF and transplant patients, too.

No one would ever write in an obituary: our dearly beloved died from bureaucratic incompetence and corporate miserliness. But if obituaries were perfectly honest, many would probably say exactly that.

We arrived at our hotel that night at two in the morning, and by the time I did treatment it was 4:30 a.m. Early the next morning my mom was up battling insurance again. I slept until noon, recovering from the stress of the day before.

When I finally woke up and started treatment again, I heard her screaming on the phone to the same low woman on the totem pole who'd been with us throughout the entire process. We had gone from thinking of her as helpful savior to corporate traitor. But that Friday, she gave us a piece of information that confirmed for us that, even if her hands were strapped behind her back, she was on our side: "Every single phone call has been recorded," she said. "You can request transcripts."

Ultimately, the woman who had been trying to help us was able to connect my mom to a higher-up at Blue Cross. We had been ringing the alarm bells for long enough that word had traveled up the food chain. My mom told her she was going to request transcripts of every single phone call, every single conversation; that my dad would take legal action if they didn't immediately grant the authorization; and that, if I couldn't be seen at UPMC the next week because I didn't have the authorization, she would be on the *Today* show first thing Monday morning to out Blue Cross for what they'd done.

During this nightmare, we discovered that a very close friend of ours is a close friend of a board member at Blue Cross. We drafted an email describing in great detail every single step of the process, and, incredibly, he said he would reach out to his contact. By the end of that long, hard first day in Pittsburgh, and after weeks of fighting, weeks of going in circles trying to get what we needed, we heard the magic words: I was approved—not just for the full evaluation, but all the way through transplant.

We don't know if my mom's threats made them change their mind, or if it was the favor called in by our incredible friend, a friend we now call our Godfather. Behind the scenes, the problem was resolved, and by Friday at 4:00 p.m. before Monday's evaluation, we knew that everything would be okay. It was as if we had been held underwater for a long time, and we could finally come up for air. It was a full-body decompression. Relief doesn't even begin to describe the feeling.

What saddens me about the situation, though, is that I do think it was our Godfather who fixed everything. It worked out beautifully for me, and I will be forever grateful for that favor; there's no way to repay a favor that could end up saving my life. But I know that others who have been in my situation, people who didn't have a hero to step in and save the day, would have gone to sleep that Friday night with no authorization; they would have had to cancel their evaluation; they would have turned around and gone home without being seen; they might have died because they couldn't get insurance approval for an evaluation or a transplant. It's not right and it needs to change. It should not be this hard for anybody.

To quote the wise words of Metallica, I just have one thing to say to Blue Cross: "Don't tread on me."

And to all people fighting insurance battles and fatal illnesses, words from high school English class (Dylan Thomas) are fitting: "Do not go gentle into that good night . . . Rage, rage, against the dying of the light."

10/12/16
I got the best birthday present ever—UPMC officially accepted me for transplant but said I'm too healthy to move to Pittsburgh

now. The evaluation had been a grueling week of meetings with doctors, surgeons, social workers, pharmacists, and financial people to make sure I met all of the criteria for transplant, and all sorts of medical tests, blood draws, imaging. It was one of the most emotionally challenging and physically difficult weeks of my life but there was a payoff!

10/31/16
Jesse sent me the lyrics to her song "Clear Lungs"!!* It's perfect:

> I may fly lower with my broken wings
> But I smile brighter every time I soar
> Sometimes I worry if I dream too big
> I will shatter like glass
> That chasing more freedom could poison the rest
>
> And I feel wasted
> And I feel tired
> And I feel lonely as I
> Watch friends disappearing
> And strain in these shackles
> That chain me to routines
> Keeping me alive
> To breathe once
> With clear lungs
> But I'm stuck on this line
>
> White masks surround me on every front
> Make me feel guilty when I want to run
> No second chances, all about percent

* "Clear Lungs" by Jesse Karlan can be heard at jessekarlan.com.

Every drop in that sign
Isolates me from a normal life

And I feel wasted
And I feel tired
And I feel lonely as I
Watch friends disappearing
And strain in these shackles
That chain me to routines
Keeping me alive
To breathe once
With clear lungs
But I'm stuck on this line

Don't wanna drown in myself
Sixty pills a day, 23 hours to health
Got this countdown running in the back of my mind
Hope for normal
Just wish for normal

I may fly lower with my broken wings
But I smile brighter every time I soar

So I'll feel wasted
And I'll feel tired
But I'll feel lucky as I
Live my life with meaning
And strive to be happy
Find beauty in the simple things
Most people fail to find
And breathe once
With clear lungs
Till I jump off this line

11/5/16

I think I need IV iron. This severe, ongoing fatigue is messing with my head.

My brain is different. I don't know if that's due to chronic lack of oxygen, but my memory is shit now, my concentration is terrible, and I've lost my ability to juggle multiple pieces of information. My processing speed is so much slower, too. That's another thing, when I'm exhausted and anemic and short of breath and high on Marinol, I don't have a gregarious personality. I kind of just recede and watch what's going on around me since it's easier not to talk, and easier to lie or sit down than to stand up. Maybe it's the mono. I think I forgot to write that they figured out that's what's been going on with me.

11/12/16

It wasn't always this way. If I was the object of others' staring in the past, I could assume it was because of my six-foot stature, so rare for a woman, people in the street would tell me. Once, in high school, I was swimming at a local community pool in Maui during spring break, trying to get back in shape for swim season in the wake of a hospitalization. A photographer there asked if he could use a photo of me swimming for a fitness magazine. I chuckled, noting the irony, but still taking my healthy appearance for granted, assuming it would last as long as I did.

For so long, while cystic fibrosis took its toll on my lungs, my pancreas, my bones, my liver, my intestines, and my stomach, the illness was invisible. It was so invisible that I could have written pieces on the difficulty of trying to get disability accommodations while looking perfectly healthy, the frustrating process of making the severity of my disease known to the skeptics on the other side of the negotiation. Those skeptics were the people who would ensure that I got through school without failing out for excessive absences and tardies; they were the people who would let me board early on airplanes, but rarely without a disapproving glare; they were the people who could either grant me the ability to work without compromising my health, or deny it.

Though having an invisible illness presents its own unique set of challenges, now I pine for the days when I could still walk down the street and blend in. I pine for the days when I could choose to hide my disease.

Now that my disease is visible, it creates walls between me and those around me. The IV pumps in my purse connected via long plastic tubing to the Mediport in my right chest are an instant spectacle. The nasal cannula connected to my oxygen tank, oxygenating my blood in ways my own body can't, is another spectacle. In short, wherever I go, I am a spectacle, and it's tiresome.

On election night, I went to a party at Talia's. There were about thirty people there, packed tight into a San Francisco apartment. People stand on their feet at these types of things; that is so hard for me, these days, even with oxygen. I meet people and I see the way their eyes jump from nasal cannula to oxygen tank to Mediport to IV tubing, the way pity swells inside of them as they realize that this is my life. I know many are wondering—does she have cancer?

There are other signs, less obvious than the equipment to which I'm tethered, perhaps noticeable only to a keen eye. The subtle thoracic kyphosis,* which worsens by the year. The edema in my ankles, a sign of mild heart failure. My disproportionately large rib cage and upper torso compared to my chicken legs and noodle arms. Clubbing, common in CF, characterized by curved and bulbous fingertips and toes. My pale skin, a trademark of the

* an excessive convex curvature of the spine

iron–deficiency anemia my doctors are too afraid to treat because iron can feed the infection in my lungs. My labored breathing, so loud it can't possibly be ignored. My periodic winces, from pleuritic chest pain or stomach cramps or migraines. The dark brown staining around my teeth, a result of the enamel being destroyed from months of frequent vomiting. The bald patches on my head, which became noticeable only after I'd become anemic and malnourished. Blue nails, deprived of oxygen. The blank look in my eyes when I can't follow a conversation because of the Marinol pills I have to take for appetite stimulation and nausea. The coughing spells that often hit when I laugh, which are painful and sometimes lead me to avoid laughter altogether.

Soon, I may have to get a feeding tube, a gastrostomy-jejunostomy tube (G-J tube). The tube bypasses the stomach and feeds liquid nutrition directly into the small intestine, ideal for patients with a lot of nausea and vomiting. I can't eat enough to keep up with my body's nutritional requirements. It will be yet another piece of medical equipment, surgically implanted into my body, just like my Mediport. It will help save my life, but it's yet another way my previously invisible illness is rendered visible.

All of these identifiers are walls that separate me from meaningful interaction with the people around me. People do not know what to say. I don't blame them; I wouldn't, either, were the roles reversed.

I pine for the days before those walls existed. I pine for the days before I had to tug my leash around, the twenty-five-foot tubing connecting me to my home oxygen machine. I pine for the days when I could play a beach volleyball match, and people would just assume I had a cough or a cold. I pine for the days when I could swim, surf, hike, even just *sit* there, *comfortably*. I pine for my invisible illness, now that it has turned visible.

11/13/16

This past week has been super hectic. Today is Sunday. On Wednesday, I went to clinic at Stanford. We discussed lots of problems: newfound swelling in my feet (possibly a sign of a blood clot, which we ruled out via ultrasound, or heart problems), continuing fevers, round-the-clock oxygen use. We talked about when to move to Pittsburgh, my weight, and their desire for me to get a G-J tube. The one thing we didn't discuss is that I think I have a partial obstruction. I wasn't as certain about it then as I am now; now I'm almost positive. At clinic I didn't want to tell them my concerns because I thought they would immediately test and treat me, which would mean an admission since I haven't been able to resolve blockages at home. And it was important to me to stay out of the hospital because the next day was Jack's birthday.

As it turns out, on his birthday I had a fever so we stayed inside while I drank hot tea and curled up with a blanket. I gave him his gifts: a North Face reversible flannel shirt-thing, Birddogs shorts (his favorite), and a framed picture of the two of us. He genuinely loved the gifts, which made me really happy.

We had a really intense conversation that night. He cried. He told me that his dad said to him, "You know this relationship is going to have a tragic ending, right?" I don't know if his dad was referring to us breaking up when Jack gets a job, or to me moving to Pittsburgh, or to the pain of watching me get sicker, or if he was talking about me dying. He could have been referring to any of those possibilities. I didn't ask because I didn't think he would want to say aloud, "He was referring to the fact that you will probably die at some point and that will be tragic because of how much I care about you."

It's at times like this that I realize how much he cares. The fact that sometimes it seems like he doesn't care is a function of com-

partmentalizing; he cares so much he can't NOT compartmentalize, otherwise he wouldn't be able to function. And to some
extent, I do the same thing. I'm not constantly tormented about
my disease; I wouldn't want him to be, either. I need to realize
that when he does not seem the most empathetic, it's not for lack
of caring but rather for lack of experience dealing with tragedy
and hardship, and an inability to figure out how to comport himself in times of crisis/sickness.

The next day was Friday. I lay low during the day except for
an interview with some people from Stanford Hospital. They're
writing a piece about me to send to donors that will appear in
their magazine. Thank God they came to Uncle Danny's house,
because I was not well enough to go out.

On Saturday, I was supposed to go out to lunch with Jack's
mom, Val. Because of my horrible night of sleep and how bad I
felt in the morning, I knew I had to change the plan. We ended
up having her over to Danny's house and my mom threw together
a small wine and appetizer party and it was really nice. Since I was
feverish, I drank tea and curled up with a blanket. And lots of
people were coming and going Aunt Lissa, Uncle Danny, cousins Sarah and Hannah, etc. It felt like a full house. Val was so nice
and not intimidating at all.

When they left, I started to feel worse. It was a really bad
evening. Spiked a high fever (I think it was above 103, but by the
time I checked, it had come down to 102.4). I felt truly horrible,
just lay there on the couch, shivering, with heating pads all over
me, drinking the hottest tea, until I fell asleep. The scariest part
was that at some point in the middle of this delirium, I felt extremely depressed and just so weary, like I couldn't go on any
longer. I thought to myself, if I'm going to feel like this, I can't
keep persisting; I can't do it anymore.

At a certain point, a person breaks. My mom is having to do

everything for me while I'm just trying to exist. I'm toxic to the people around me and my body is toxic to myself. I thought about what it would be like to just not exist anymore. Not to kill myself, obviously; I would never do that. But I just thought, *What if I did have some kind of heart problem and just went to sleep and didn't wake up?* That thought was even more stressful to me than the idea of living with sickness because of what it would do to my family.

So I will persist. But something needs to change, something needs to improve, if not with my actual health, then at least with my palliative care to keep me more comfortable as I struggle. Marinol is a good first step, but I'm sure there are other things that could be helping.

12/1/16
Need to write about what happened after reaching the glorious acceptance by UPMC. A viral infection pushed me off the summit. I free-fell into the deepest abyss of illness I've ever faced. A spate of complications drove me to panic: severe fatigue (which fourteen hours of sleep a night couldn't reckon with), complete loss of appetite, incessant nausea and vomiting, respiratory distress with any amount of exertion, and oxygen saturations plummeting into the 70s when I changed clothes or walked to the bathroom (they are supposed to stay above 90 at all times). When I went to the emergency room on October 28, I collapsed in the waiting room walking to the check-in desk. A week later, when I got discharged, I hardly felt better.

Then Jack's b'day, which I wrote about.

Then Sabrina came to visit from Philadelphia, and I spent most of the time asleep. I accrued more worrisome symptoms: strange lumps that I worried were tumors and swelling of the legs and ankles (edema with pitting). My heart thrashed around inside my chest, feeling like a fish trying to escape a fisherman's hook.

Stanford told me to come in for an echocardiogram, which showed mild heart failure. They wanted to admit me right then, that Monday before Thanksgiving, and told me I should not plan on going home (which meant I'd miss both Thanksgiving and Mallory's Garden). Thanksgiving is my favorite holiday and I was desperate to be at the fundraiser so my mom suggested we call UCLA and ask for a direct admit—which Dr. Eshaghian was willing to arrange. We left straight from the echo test at Stanford, flew to L.A., and then my dad picked us up and took us straight to a room at UCLA Medical Center in Santa Monica, bypassing the ER.

I spent the week there but was discharged in time for our twenty-first annual CF fundraiser. There, we announced our departure and said emotional goodbyes to our community. But then, three days later, we got another call from the coordinator at Pittsburgh, explaining that the team there had changed their mind. Once they put all the pieces together in their transplant meeting—the mono, the heart problems, the timeline of my decline—they realized that if mono was causing most of these problems, then when the mono went away, I might be too healthy to be ready for transplant. They did not want me to move all the way to Pittsburgh just to get healthy again a month later and have to turn around and go home.

More important, they couldn't list me for transplant with mild heart failure without listing me for a heart AND lung transplant. No one wanted to do that, since I had a perfectly healthy heart up until I contracted the mono. The Pittsburgh doctor's decision was that I should wait until the mono cleared and until the heart function improved; at that point, we would determine if it was still the right time for me to be listed.

By the time I heard the news of their change of heart, two days before Thanksgiving, I'd ridden an emotional roller coaster trying to come to terms with the idea of moving to Pittsburgh.

And I finally had. In fact, I'd done such a good job of coming to terms with it that when I found out they'd changed their mind, I was devastated; I'd actually wanted to go to Pittsburgh, I realized. In order to get better, in order to get a transplant and live the life I want to live, I have to get worse. I have to pay my dues. I have to move to Pittsburgh. I was ready for that next step. But it was a false alarm.

12/2/16

I feel like people with CF are privy to secrets it takes most other people a lifetime to understand. How lucky we are to be alive. How lucky anyone is who has their health. How we should be appreciative of anything that's in our control since our health is not. That we can leave behind a legacy when we go that will impact others. That simple things are often the most beautiful. That love and happiness are the most important things to strive for. That ultimately, we shouldn't give a damn what other people think, because everyone's making their own way and everyone's facing different struggles that others aren't aware of. CF has given me my value system and ultimately, no matter how hard it is, I'm grateful for it.

12/3/16

New Year's is important to me. Not New Year's Eve; I've never liked that night as far as holidays go. But the new year and the weeks leading up to New Year's always force me into a state of reflection that I generally don't get to at any other time.

So as the new year approaches, I find myself reflecting. This year has been monumental. Colossal. As far as change goes, who I am and what my plans are for the future changed weekly this year, whereas in the past, they changed over the course of months or years. My resilience has been challenged and my ability to adapt has been called upon. "Mind over matter" has never been more important.

Questions that have been prominent: those of identity; what matters to me now and in the future; who matters to me now and in the future; how I can keep my mind stimulated while my body deteriorates; how I can accept the fact that my body is deteriorating; how I can be happy while feeling like absolute shit.

I don't have the answers. It's a struggle. There have been many low points. But I realize that as time goes on, what I define as a low point will keep changing. For example, at UCLA hospital in January, I was traumatized by having to use the toilet inside the fishbowl of the ICU room. I demanded to walk to the bathroom in the hallway each time I had to go, which was frequently, because I drink so much water. When I was too sick or unstable to walk to the bathroom, it felt like defeat. It was crushing, humiliating, and dehumanizing. Now, in my most recent hospitalization (again at UCLA—coming full circle this year despite lots of Stanford admissions in between), I requested a bedside commode because I literally couldn't bring myself to walk the five extra steps to the bathroom in my room. I voluntarily embraced the bedside toilet, something that a year ago was unfathomable to me. I call this progress.

It's sad that I have to come to terms with these things, but transplant is going to test me in ways I can't even imagine now. Being on a ventilator in the ICU and having to have my butt wiped in the bed by some male nurse assistant is going to be my reality, either pre-transplant or post. There will be pain beyond what I can tolerate right now. I only hope my pain tolerance adapts and that I don't wilt under the force of all the hardship.

Another thing to get used to is my diminishing brain power. I used to be smart. I didn't know what it would be like to be less smart—but now I do. I don't remember things. I don't draw connections in the way that I used to. I don't understand complex concepts. I can't focus on books, and thus I've lost an entire world I used to have as an escape. Not one world—many worlds. Being smart was a part of my identity that I took for granted because I didn't think that would change. I heard a quote recently about books that was something like, "Though I remember nothing of the plots of the books I've read, nonetheless, they've made me." And that is so true. Books have taught me compassion. They've taught me to see beyond the bubble I was raised in. They've shown me other experiences, other lives, other worlds. They've awakened in me a spirit of adventure, which now lies dormant. They're like friends that I've pushed away, but now I miss them.

12/8/16

Today was my first day of pulmonary rehab at UCLA. It inspired me to take more action to control what I can with my health. And where that starts is with exercise (and nutrition, but I'm already working on that).

I feel like my body is a foreign object, one I don't understand. The CF rules I've learned my whole life and biology I learned in school do not apply, because something more complicated is going on.

I'm giving myself a goal and that's to be able to walk on the beach on hard sand for twenty minutes by the time Jack comes and we go to Malibu. I just have to have something concrete to work toward or I will languish.

In some ways, I struggle so much more than any twenty-four-year-old deserves to. But in some ways, I'm privileged beyond belief. I wish those two things canceled out to make me feel somewhat normal. Instead, I just feel the deepest lows of CF misery, and the incredibly fortunate highs of having the family and friends and resources to live as well as possible despite that. Having

the most incredible house in Malibu offered to us by Walter and
Hildy for Christmas vacation? Unreal. It's unbelievable. Having
Jan buy me a really great coat for the Pittsburgh winter, even
though we're probably not even going this winter anymore? Also
unreal. I just have to do my best to keep those feelings of gratitude
at the forefront. And that's easy when I'm feeling well; it comes
naturally to my healthy self. But it's like I have a split personality.
When I feel sick, everything feels terrible, and my future feels so
bleak, and I can't stand the idea of being around anyone, and I
can't stand the idea of being alone—it's a catch-22 that leaves me
stuck in a trap of unhappiness, which I recognize from the outside
as being absurd, but it's like a nightmare I can't wake up from.
While I'm in it, I don't have the ability to change the channel
away from self-pity so I can only do my best while I am healthy(ish)
to bolster my sick self through the sick times by coming up with
strategies to remind myself of how lucky I am, even when I feel
like absolute shit. When I feel good the world is filled with endless possibilities.

I'm so conflicted about whether to stay in L.A. or go back to
S.F. in January. There are pros and cons to each.

LOS ANGELES:

Pros: time with family and Maria and Kona, being well-fed all
the time, warm weather, less pressure to be social and more time
to rest, amazing adjustable bed where I can raise the head, which
helps me sleep. L.A. is comfortable. All my stuff is here so it's the
path that inertia leads me to. I can go to the beach and put my
feet in the water. I can be treated at UCLA, with all the personal
attention and nurturing qualities of Dr. Eshaghian.

Cons: don't want to lose touch with my S.F. friends;
wouldn't get to see Jack very much; don't know how much longer I get to live in California so maybe I should be acting like a

twentysomething-year-old by being in my own apartment, surrounded by friends.

If I go back to S.F., am I going to have enough help? Am I
going to be lonely being in my apartment by myself, or, on the
opposite end of the spectrum, will I feel smothered by hanging
out with my mom? Is it just going to remind me of all the things
I can't do, now that I'm wearing O_2 24/7 and don't feel super
comfortable or stoked about going out at night?

SAN FRANCISCO:

Pros: get to see Jack and friends all the time. The light filtering
in through my window, through which I see the ocean and the
Golden Gate Bridge. My desk, organization, the feeling of pro-
ductivity I have there. The gym. My old routines. Feeling like
I'm living out my S.F. life for as long as I possibly can.

Cons: thirty-two stairs to get up to my apartment, and hills to
walk anytime I want to go anywhere. Less help. No one to cook
for me. Cold weather. I have to be treated at Stanford, where it's
difficult to get what you need unless you're an inpatient. Pressure
to get feeding tube from Stanford team. Possibility of Jack leaving
soon after I move back, if he gets a job on the East Coast.

So conflicted.

The main thing I worry about up there is loneliness. But it's
funny because the main thing I worry about in L.A. is also loneliness. CF is just an isolating disease but I don't do anything to try
to combat that; I just get tired and watch TV alone. I think I
would benefit from therapy but I don't go. Except that there's no
one else to talk about my issues *with*—other CF patients deal with
their own issues and it's really hard to complain to people who are
worse off, and those who are better off don't understand; healthy
friends don't understand and often don't say the right thing. They
say things like, "I'm sure it will be fine," "I'm sure you'll get bet-

ter," "Stay positive," all platitudes that don't really help. With Jack, for some reason it just doesn't feel natural talking about my problems; I minimize things. It kills my mom to see me sad so I don't want to burden her with that when she and my dad are going through their own struggles as my caretakers.

I'm starting to think therapy is the only option because in my own head I just go in circles, and with others, it's not working well. And I need to be so mentally strong before transplant. I need to be at peace with the idea of death while also fiercely wanting to live; it's hard to feel both at the same time.

Anyway, back to pulmonary rehab. They want me to walk six minutes, three times a day. I think if I do that I can build up to walking twenty minutes on the beach. That plus the resistance/weight stuff I'm doing with my trainer should help me and maybe put on a couple pounds of muscle—then I can get the dietitians off my back.

12/22/16

Wednesday morning, I woke up to tragic news— a blog post by Caitlin's mom (the girl I met when I was in Pittsburgh for my evaluation). They had been there for two and a half years waiting for transplant. She worked so hard and did everything right. But then her health crashed, and she ended up on life support (ECMO and ventilator). She was having all sorts of problems and I was following the updates from her mom on the blog. Because I've been working on David's memoir, I have more insight into transplant than I otherwise would. And as I saw how sick she was getting, I kept wondering if Stanford would have already removed her from the transplant list for being too sick. But UPMC didn't, and after a couple of dry runs with lungs that weren't viable, she finally got lungs, perfect lungs.

But she was still in critical condition. They couldn't close her chest because of swelling, and even though Maryanne made it seem on the blog like that was normal, I knew that if they cannot close the chest, the likelihood of the patient making it is slim. She was having more problems though, her blood pressure was too low, she had rising lactate levels, which signified dead tissue somewhere, and they didn't know if it was in her leg or her liver or her bowel. And her liver started to fail, and maybe her kidneys, too.

The next day I read that she had died. It was devastating. I immediately started bawling and could not control myself. I let myself cry for ten or fifteen minutes, thinking about her family, thinking about how hard she fought, and how futile it all turned out to be. All that struggle, all that uprooting, and now she's just dead. Gone forever. It felt like my heart was being squeezed by a vise grip.

12/28/16
I find myself thinking about Caitlin, her family, and how tragic her ending was. It reminds me to be grateful for the health I do have.

12/31/16
My anniversary card to Jack:

Jack,

I can't believe a year has come and gone already. When I met you on NYE 2015/2016, I never could've guessed that you would become one of the most important people in my life, in one of the most important times of my life. I'm so lucky to be with you—you're caring, smart, funny, so fun to be around, so handsome, and so, so, so good to me. Ever since the day you charmed my grandparents—two weeks into our relationship—I knew you were a keeper! Time and again, though, you've surprised me with your willingness to jump into this crazy life of mine. It amazes me, but it also doesn't, because you're amazing. I know this distance thing we're doing is hard, and we don't know what will happen in the future. But whatever does happen, I want to thank you deeply for an incredible year with you and for the best relationship I've ever had. Paradise really is anywhere I'm with you (although I do hope for more times in true paradisiacal places in the future) :) Love you so much.

Mal

2017

1/24/17

In the hospital at UCLA Santa Monica. Been struggling with the usual symptoms.

We are likely going to Pittsburgh in two weeks. Mom started crying today when she talked to Dr. Eshaghian about the fact that then she has to leave me to go to S.F. to pack up my apartment, and then we're going to Pitt soon after that. It made me so sad to see her cry. She always puts up such a tough and strong front, but I know that there's so much sadness and fear underneath that she rarely lets anyone see.

1/26/17

Today is a better day. My lungs are clearing out and I didn't wake up at 6:00 to bring up floods of mucus. I'm no longer using morphine for shortness of breath or lung pain. And I'm not having fevers, which is the other biggest thing!! The fevers would prevent me from being listed because it would show that we don't have the infection under control. Pitt wants them under control.

Sounds like we're going to Pitt in five days to a week. Wouldn't be surprised if it was end of next week, which would be ironic because I think a few people are coming to town to see me that weekend. Don't remember, though, because my memory is shit.

2/10/17

The past week was hellish. I kept spontaneously bursting into tears. Talia had a going-away party for me on Wednesday night so I could say my goodbyes at one time instead of trying to see everyone separately. There was so much back-and-forth about me going/not going/going/not going so in the end, I only had two days at home between when I got out of the hospital and when I had to be across the country for UPMC's clinic. It was stressful trying to pack up my entire life to move across the country while 1) battling end-stage lung disease with fevers and an acute infection, 2) spending my last two days with Jack before being long-distance, 3) saying goodbye to my grandparents, who will be dead most likely when I'm back, 4) saying goodbye to my dog, which feels like abandoning my own child, and 5) saying goodbye to Maria.

Yesterday, I took the biggest leap of my life into the scariest chapter of my life. UPMC has given me reason to hope. Dr. Pilewski is my hero for being willing to gamble on high-risk cases like mine—and for giving me a second chance at life.

I left California so I don't become a life-expectancy statistic or a sad case study written about in a medical paper. I left to chase the dream of a better and longer future. A four-hour flight across the country was the beginning of the journey. My mom, dad, Linda, and Dr. Monvasi, a doctor from Tampa that David recommended, flew with me. It was the last nonstop American flight from L.A. to Pittsburgh before they discontinued the route. It was so nice to have help moving.

I still can't believe we're in Pittsburgh for good (temporarily for good, oxymoronic as that may be).

2/13/17

JUST GOT THE CALL THAT I'M LISTED!!! I was in bed at our hotel taking a nap, then woke up and was on the phone with Sabrina. Got a call from a 412 number and should have answered but ignored it because I hadn't talked to Sab in so long and didn't want to cut her off. Then two mins later my mom comes busting in with the biggest smile on her face, on the phone, and tells me that it was UPMC and that I was listed!!

We thought the call might come tomorrow but I didn't want to get my hopes up. And then it came early! Such a relief. But it also means we're now on call 24/7 so I can never turn my phone off again and I should have a hospital bag packed so that I'm always ready.

It's surreal.

Stanford had said that no one would give me a transplant but now UPMC is doing something miraculous. I don't think it ever really sank in that I WOULDN'T get a transplant, but there was enough doubt to know that this is a huge moment. Huge huge huge moment!

Right after I got the call, Jack texted me to pick up his FaceTime and I did and then my mom brought in a bouquet of a dozen roses. They were from Jack for Valentine's Day!

2/18/17

The past few days have been okay. We rode the high of me getting listed for a couple of days, which was great, before settling back into our new normal. It could take months or a year or more to get the call, so we have to straddle the line to be ready at any moment but also prepared for a long wait. It's a bit of a mind fuck.

The thing that scares me is my persistent fevers. If I got the call today, what would I say? Whenever I don't take Tylenol or Advil on the dot of six hours, I start getting chills and a fever. I don't know how high it would go, because I'm continually suppressing. I can't go into surgery with active infection. But I ALWAYS have active infection, which is why I need to be on IVs.

Caitlin's mom and dad are in Pittsburgh to pack up for their move back to Boston. They did what we did—moved here to get listed since their own hospital in Boston wouldn't transplant Caitlin because of *cepacia*. They invited us to a party given by their neighbors. It was a chance to say goodbye to all the people they'd gotten to know in the two and a half years they were here.

I was going to go but wasn't feeling well so my mom went without me. After the Advil and Tylenol kicked in, I finished treatment and was hungry so wanted to get dinner. We were still in a hotel so I texted my mom to find out if she had eaten. She asked if I wanted to come to the party and so I went. Everyone was so nice, especially the hosts, Ralph and Mary. My dad had already gone back to L.A. so my mom was ecstatic to make friends in a city where she knew no one. And everyone was so welcoming and sweet.

It was tragic to see Maryanne and Nick. Apparently my mom was crying when she arrived and Nick (Caitlin's dad) gave her a stern talking-to, basically saying something like, "We're not doing this. You have one job now, and that's to take care of Mallory. You have to be on it, and right now you're a blubbering mess."

When I arrived and looked at him sadly, he said (very nicely), "We're not going to do this, I already told your mom." He was so nice and gave me Caitlin's old oxygen carrier that she made with her boyfriend. I think Maryanne was having a harder time by the end, and she did cry when she said goodbye to us. I didn't know what to do, what to say, how to act. That was why I was worried about going in the first place, because they're grieving the loss of their daughter while I represent the beginning of the journey, and what are they supposed to say? "I hope it goes better for you than it did for Caitlin"? They did basically say that. She said, "I'm so happy you're even taller than I remember. You're not going to have to wait like Caitlin did—she was too small to receive most donor lungs."

I'm happy I went. Ralph and Mary invited us back again on Sunday for a pasta party, and we're going to go. Stacy will be here then to help my mom move us into the new apartment. Today is our last day at the Fairmont so I'm going to try to muster the energy to foam roll at the gym and use the sauna, just to take advantage of it for the one last day.

2/28/17

Since I last wrote, every single day (until yesterday and today) I had a fever pattern that was the same every day. I would start shivering madly around 1:00 p.m., after Tylenol and Advil, and as the fever went up I would feel like shit—shortness of breath, tachycardia up to 140 bpm at rest, nausea, the works—and then the fever would spike up to 102 or 103, or some days even higher (one day it got to 103.7), then it would go down. When the fever would finally break, around 4:00 or 5:00 or 6:00, my appetite would come back in full force and I would eat a ton to make up for having not eaten for hours.

This pattern was unsettling. I kept thinking we should tell

Larry, my transplant coordinator. The day I spiked up to 103.7
I packed my bag for the ER; it did not occur to me in my
wildest dreams that they would tell me to stay home. But they
did! And then a few days later—Sunday, to be specific—I just
didn't have a fever that day. I was exhausted, for sure, but no
fever. It was miraculous. It might've been the right call not to
go to the ER, but the day I called I was so anxious. I was bawling in bed and thought things were going to end in tragedy for
me and for my family. I was terrified. The fevers reduce me to
this scared, shriveled, sick, anxious blubberer with no sense of
control over any part of my future. The fevers are the hardest
thing for me right now. When the fevers are gone, life feels
manageable.

I need a long-term kind of project to occupy myself with
while I'm here. Maybe take up a musical instrument? Or start my
book? That's what my mom thinks I should do but not sure I'm
up for that yet. I guess it can't hurt to brainstorm.

Oh, to dream about what it could be like . . . it makes me
wilt a bit. To think about all the girls who, in the exact same
position that I'm in now, were filled with so much hope, and
dreamt about all they would do post-transplant, working so
hard to stay alive to get to that goal, who then didn't make it in
the end. Caitlin, I think of her so often. Her mom sent me a
blog post that Caitlin wrote where so much of it hit close to
home about the experience of coming to terms with being
listed for transplant and coming to recognize it as a beautiful
opportunity to have so much GREATER of a life than what
we've had for years. It made me want to cry, though, because
she wrote it only about a year before she died, and she had no
idea how terribly it would all turn out. No one did. It wasn't
fair. And it won't be fair if it happens to me. Transplant scares
the shit out of me.

3/5/17

I never wrote about Bakery Living! It's the apartment my mom and I live in here in Pittsburgh. It's amazing and cozy. The lobby is like a hotel with coffee every day and bagels on the weekends. They have a gym we work out in and monthly activities that create community. Freddie and Samir are the first two people I met.

3/28/17

Had another massive bleed. I need new lungs. Apparently the amount of hemoptysis I had this time has a 50 to 85 percent mortality rate without embolization. I just keep wondering what happens if the bleeding doesn't stop in time for them to embolize. Last night, lying in bed, I found myself replaying the scene in the ER but with an alternate ending. I pictured the bleeding going and going and not stopping until I lost consciousness and my pressures dropped and I inhaled the blood and then died. And I mainly just pictured my mom and dad crying, and it made me cry just thinking that that could have happened.

4/3/17

A girl, a CF patient, who was treated at Stanford, Monica Harding Wood, died sometime this weekend. Or at least I found out this weekend. She had been completely fine and her death came out of nowhere. She had advanced disease and was close to being listed for transplant, but she was totally stable and there was no indication that she was near the end. She went in for a port placement and G-J tube procedure and somehow died in the process, no idea how. It's so tragic and so terrifying.

My mom went to L.A. last week to be with my grandma. She comes back today and my dad leaves tomorrow. I'll miss him a lot. But I do think it will be good to have my mom here again because she does things for me and for the apartment that I don't have to ask her to do. The apartment is always clean, I get three meals a day, there are always groceries, the laundry gets done frequently, etc. Pidge needs more sleep, plus he has to work for his job. He just doesn't move as quickly as she does (no one does) so not as much gets done. But it was SO nice to have him here, to be able to spend quality time together. We watched movies, talked about books, and had a lot of good meals. I'm sad he's leaving.

My mom is bringing our new dog tonight!! I'm hoping and choosing to believe that having Cooper here will turn things around for me emotionally at a time where I could either go back to "normal" or fall off an emotional cliff.

4/7/17

Cooper is so cute but has issues. He was a rescue and my mom learned AFTER she brought him home that he'd been returned three times. Hoping we can get him to calm down and feel safe. I already love him. . . .

4/21/17

The day started out the way mornings have been starting out for the last few weeks: with fatigue, nausea, an attempt at breakfast, vomiting, some chills, nausea meds and fever suppression, and thoughts about a nap. But Talia was in town, and I was determined to make the day a good day.

I was doing my breathing treatments in my bedroom while she was having breakfast in the living room. My mom was out walking the dog. The phone rang with the Pittsburgh area code, 412. When we first moved to Pittsburgh in February, I would always jump at those calls, thinking they were about lungs; eventually, when time and again they were just hospital administrators confirming appointments, the home health nurse, or medication refills, I stopped getting my hopes up.

"Hello?" I said.

"Hi, Mallory, this the Cardiothoracic Transplant Program at UPMC."

My heart started to beat faster. The Cardiothoracic Transplant Program does not usually call me.

"I'm calling because we have a potential set of lungs available for you. But I have to ask. Are you willing to consider lungs that are on EVLP?"

I immediately said yes. EVLP, which stands for *ex vivo* lung perfusion, is an investigational procedure/machine used to keep lungs in good shape while they're transported from the donor to the recipient. Not everyone says yes to lungs that are on EVLP because it's new(ish) and experimental, but for me, it was an automatic yes. On EVLP, lungs can be manipulated to better determine their quality, and keeping the lungs perfused with the machine can prevent swelling or other complications that would render them nonviable for donation.

The woman said she would call back in an hour or so with more information. As soon as I hung up with her, I dialed my mom and yelled into the phone that I got the call. "What call?" she asked. "THE CALL!!"

Talia stood by me as I started crying, feeling the implications of this moment all at once. My mom came bursting into the apartment frenzied, tears in her eyes. By 4:00 p.m., we got the go-ahead to pack up and get to the hospital. By 5:00 p.m., we were in registration, watching TV and making silly videos to pass the time until we could get into our room.

There are many points along the way after getting the call for lungs at which the surgery can be called off. We had always known that at any point from the death of the donor to the time they remove the lungs of the recipient, surgery can be called off because the lungs are not good enough.

After a short wait in registration, I was put into a room on 9D, the lung transplant floor. Two nurses collected seventeen vials of blood—blood type and screen, as well as a slew of tests to determine whether I was healthy enough to undergo surgery. One tech came to do a bedside chest X-ray, and another came for an EKG. They took vitals, my weight, a urine sample. At that point, we settled in for the long wait.

We were itching for someone to come talk to us who could give us more information about the viability of the lungs and the timing. Finally, a cardiothoracic surgical fellow, a mellow Chilean man, arrived. He told us that the "donor time" was set for 2:00 a.m. However, the donor was in a category called DCD (Donation after Cardiac Death); this means that he or she did not meet formal brain death criteria but had suffered irreversible brain injury and was near death. The family had decided to discontinue life support systems; once that happened, they would wait for the heart to stop beating. Only after cardiac arrest would organs be harvested. When the dying process takes more than about an hour, the lungs become nonviable, because as the body struggles, the lungs can become damaged. DCD lungs are often (maybe always) put on EVLP in order to improve quality and increase the chances that the lungs can be transplanted. But the likelihood of a transplant actually happening from a DCD donor is a bit lower than from a typical donor that meets criteria for brain death.

Listening to the fellow explain what would happen at 2:00 a.m. at the donor hospital—the pulling of the plug, the waiting to die, then the eventual harvesting of organs—I was struck by the two completely different experiences that were happening at the same exact time. One family undergoing heartbreak they would forever grieve. Another family celebrating the possible rebirth of a sick loved one who has suffered too long. The first person's tragedy had the potential to become the second person's lifesaving miracle.

My survival is dependent on the death of someone else, another human being with memories and goals and loved ones and, often, no expectation of dying. This is the twisted reality of being on the waiting list. How do we, as transplant patients, come to terms with the idea of "waiting" for someone to die, with hoping it happens quickly enough for the organs to be allocated and not wasted? I expect I will grapple with this question for years to come.

When I got summoned to the hospital by the cardiothoracic department, we called Gaby to come. She was in D.C. so it was a quick flight. Throughout that evening and overnight, Talia, Gaby, and my mom helped keep me calm when my nerves were practically bursting through the seams. I was a wreck of wired, restless energy and tempered hope. At some point, Talia and my mom left to go sleep at the apartment while Gaby got comfortable in the (terribly uncomfortable) recliner chair that so many hospitals carry for guests to sleep in. I suspected I wouldn't sleep a wink, I was right.

For hours, Gaby and I sat there chatting, laughing, passing the time. It felt like two girls having a sleepover. It did not feel like we were in a hospital—I was not hooked up to an IV pole or a heart monitor, no nurses were coming in and out, no vitals were being taken by a nurse's aide, and no medications or breathing treatments were given. We just waited and waited but no news.

I finally turned off the lights and rolled over to try to sleep but it wasn't happening. I lay there, thinking, wondering what was happening at the donor hospital, what the timing would be, when they would tell us if the surgery was a go or not. I checked the clock every ten minutes until I realized that if I didn't turn on a movie, I'd crash and burn from adrenaline by the morning. My neck and back ached, and I had rock-sized knots in my back, neck, and shoulders from the tension.

I had thought that at around 4:00 a.m. they would come in

and tell me whether the lungs were looking viable. Four a.m. came and went, as did 5:00, 6:00, and 7:00. Alarms and code announcements outside the room jolted me awake any time I got close to falling asleep (the "Condition F" fire alarm seemed to last forever and was immediately followed up by a "Condition A"—cardiac arrest). The sun came up. I mixed and infused my morning IV antibiotics. I was fatigued, my optimism waning. I called for respiratory therapy to administer a breathing treatment, to help with the chest tightness and cough that had been doing its part in keeping me up.

Then, at 7:30 a.m., a man came to my room with a gurney to tell me he was taking me to the pre-op area. "Does that mean the surgery's happening?!"

"As far as I know, it's on," the guy said. "But I'm not the one who would know."

"That's abrupt," I said.

In the pre-op area, I finally found out some details about the timing from the anesthesiologist. The lungs, at that point, were still on EVLP and would need one to two more hours of manipulation to determine if they were viable. While we waited, he talked to us in detail about the anesthesia during the surgery, the sedation post-surgery, and a bit about the difficulty and risks of the surgery itself. He assured me that they would not bring me out from sedation after surgery until they were certain that I would not be in pain—this was very comforting to me, because the idea of being hooked to a ventilator and possibly ECMO, in pain, immobile, and unable to speak, was unfathomable.

Jack had been in Boston for the past week for a conference, so he got on a 6:00 a.m. flight to Pittsburgh to try to see me before I went into surgery. He arrived around 9:00, in time to hear some of the conversation with the anesthesiologist.

Finally, we met the man we've been waiting to meet ever

since my first evaluation in Pittsburgh last October, Dr. D'Cunha. He is the head transplant surgeon with the most amazing reputation. Unfortunately, he came in that morning to tell us that the lungs were good but *someone else* was going into surgery. I'm happy for that other person, but it came as a complete shock.

What we did not know until this moment was that UPMC will sometimes call in two patients for the same set of lungs to ensure that they don't get wasted. If they only called in one patient per set and then the lungs didn't end up being a good fit (because of size or other reasons), it would be a tragic waste of precious organs that too many people die waiting for.

I had assumed that once I'd made it to the pre-op area, I was the only candidate for the particular set of lungs that had just been harvested. What I found out later is that the entire time, those many hours of waiting, I was actually the backup candidate, which would have been helpful to know at the beginning (for the purpose of managing expectations).

The only good thing about the experience is that we got to meet Dr. D'Cunha. The stakes had been high, emotions fraying, nerves unraveling. When he told us I wasn't getting the lungs, it was like he stuck a needle into an overfilled balloon of anticipatory stress. I was sad that I wouldn't be getting my rebirth that day, but also a little bit relieved that I wouldn't have to be sawed open down the chest just yet.

When my mom asked how I was feeling about it all as we left the pre-op area, my answer was: "Definitely disappointed. But also a little relieved. Mainly starving. Can we go to Starbucks?"

Those twenty-one hours, from 1:00 p.m. Friday to 10:00 a.m. Saturday, were emotional, crazy, and definitely hazy. My anxiety levels have never swung so wildly, so quickly. But my crew of First Responders—my mom, Talia, and Gaby there that first day and Jack the second—eased the bumpiness of the roller-coaster

ride that it was. After the hospital, we left and got Turkish food at
11:00 a.m. Warm bread and olives, soft-boiled eggs, halvah, jams,
Turkish coffee, kebabs of various meats and rice, and pickled cabbage and salads, all after a day of fasting and an all-nighter, have a
way of soothing the heart and providing some distance from the
disappointment.

Sunday morning rolled around. Jack left. Talia and Gaby and
I planned a normal day, hanging around in the morning and then
going to lunch in the afternoon. At 4:00 p.m., in the car on the
way home from lunch, I got another call from the Cardiothoracic
Transplant Program, from the same person who had called me on
Friday. There was another set of lungs for me, I was told, and this
time, there were no other recipients being called. The donor was
not DCD, and the surgeons were not planning on using EVLP on
the lungs. This sounded super promising, and she said to get to
the hospital quickly. It was more stressful this time because my
mom had been sick and vomiting the entire day—probably from
stress and exhaustion—but we made it to the hospital in a much
shorter time frame since my bag was still packed from the previous trip two days prior. After getting to the hospital at 5:00 p.m.
Sunday evening and waiting in the ER for five hours before getting registered, by 2:00 a.m. we were in pre-op, and a surgeon was
coming to tell us that the lungs had been deemed nonviable in the
donor surgery. After two and a half months of no calls, in one
weekend I got two calls that turned out to be two dry runs.

Two dry runs in one weekend is absurdly comical for someone who's healthy enough to wait a bit longer, like I am. But for
those who are at the very end, who might not live another day or
another week or another month, having more people signed up
to be organ donors is the difference between life and death. My
friend Caitlin fell on the wrong side of that divide, simply because
she had to wait too damn long to get lungs, and by the time she

did (almost three years after being listed), her body had just been through too much. My heart still breaks for her family.

This process is crazy. And exciting. After a weekend of sleeplessness, I have nothing profound to say about it. My sentiments can be summed up by: holy shit. Here's hoping the third time's the charm.

5/3/17

I feel good about things. I've had a good feeling the past few days. Maybe because things are so good with Jack. I have the strength and stamina to walk around with my O_2 backpack, which makes me SO much more mobile and independent and makes me feel like my recovery would be quicker if I got the transplant in this current condition. I like that I have a steady stream of friends visiting, with at least a day break in between. I feel so loved.

I'm really sad about my grandparents, though. They are not doing well. My mom's voice sounds so grave on the phone (she's back in L.A. cuz it's the end with her mom) and she's eager to hang up, which is not her normal. I miss Grandma already and she's not even dead yet—but this is what I knew would happen. I knew I wouldn't really be able to keep in touch with them from afar because Grandma would get so sick. Now Grandpa is in a ton of pain from a fall, but his needs are kind of secondary to hers so I think his pain is not really being addressed. It's all terrible.

5/5/17

Grandma died today. I don't really have words; I've been feeling run-down all week but all the symptoms really hit me hard today, and that, combined with the complicated emotional experience of grief, has left me completely drained. I can barely muster the energy to talk out loud.

I don't really know how to grieve her and honor her memory when I couldn't be there with her at the end. I don't know if there will be a funeral but regardless, I can't go. It just feels unnatural, like tomorrow will come around and I'll forget about it until something reminds me of her and I will have to remember that she's gone.

My mom flew back to be with me last night, Aunt Meryl was with Grandma and called to say it was the end, so my mom spoke to Grandma on speaker. It was sweet to listen to; they talked about memories of her, said they loved her and would miss her but that everyone would be okay. My mom was on the couch having this conversation, and I was at the kitchen table, bawling my eyes out.

After Grandma died, my mom jumped into action. But she was crying, so I hugged her. I feel powerless to help and guilty that my mom flew back here last night and missed the actual end. My mom said Grandma wanted her to be with me so I guess I understand.

We spent a long time going through photos of Grandma and family to find ones for my mom to post on Facebook. I helped a lot with that.

5/13/17

On Monday I had a call with a Penn med student who is writing a story for *Slate,* about gender and wait times for organ transplants. Apparently, women wait longer. I hope to continue advocating for the issues surrounding transplantation.

Jack left for Europe on Thursday with his mom. His Wi-Fi on the riverboat is shitty so between that and the time change I don't expect we'll talk much over the next couple of weeks. It'll feel weird to not catch up at the end of each day. I've gotten used to that.

I got a Fitbit gift in the mail yesterday! It was a great surprise from Emily. She is SO thoughtful.

5/21/17

Things have been pretty good lately, all things considered. Stable!! Went to see Dr. Pilewski in clinic last week and didn't have much to talk about, which is a first! I LOVE him and the three women he works with.

Jeremiah and Marla got married this weekend in Cleveland, and I went! Micah and Dad flew in from L.A. so the four of us could drive to Cleveland together. First family trip without friends or boyfriends or girlfriends in literally YEARS—maybe even a decade? It was nice to spend the alone time with Micah. I feel like we never really got quality time together when I came to L.A. from NorCal because we were always in big groups or with people we were dating or at large dinners. So it was nice to have sibling time and actually catch up on each other's lives.

The wedding was so nice, the bride's family is one of the nicest families I think I've ever met. The whole weekend was amazing but EXHAUSTING. My dad and Micah flew back to L.A. so it was just my mom and me once we got home.

My mom was unpacking for hours. Crazy how much stuff I have to travel with. I couldn't sleep so I decided to get up and try the ukulele Micah brought from L.A. It had been a gift I got him three years ago but he said he'd be happy to lend it to me. I did a deep Internet search about ukulele basics, chords, simple songs to play, and listened to some Bruddah Iz songs a couple of times through. The first was "Take Me Home, Country Road" and the second was "Somewhere Over the Rainbow," although I really struggled with that one. My mom always sings, "Somewhere over the rainbow, there are lungs." She says it keeps her optimistic.

5/25/17

I'm in the hospital. I coughed up lots of blood on Tuesday, the day after coming home from the wedding. At 4:00 p.m. I had a big bleed that led me to call an ambulance, but the small bleeds had started at 2:00 a.m. I'm thankful that the bleeding didn't continue and that they didn't have to embolize. Knock on wood.

Today has been hard. Things started out badly when my mom heard from the transplant coordinator that Dr. Hayanga, the surgeon we met with during the eval, is leaving to start up a new transplant center in West Virginia. The volume of transplants will go down, but I didn't realize how much this news affected her until she recounted the information on the phone to my dad and started crying. She seems like she's losing it a bit, between hearing this news, the hospital staff giving her shit yesterday for blocking the door while I took a nap (then ratting her out to Dr. Pilewski), and the pharmacy staff messing up my meds. Normally, she handles so much without cracking that I don't know what pushed her over the edge this time. It could've been the hemoptysis (bigger than usual), or maybe it's the aftermath of grief from her mom dying, or maybe it's sleeplessness. All I know is she seems down.

I get it. Transplant scares the shit out of me, so for the first time in my life I'm choosing to be ignorant rather than research what's to come so I can prepare myself. I don't want to know about the vent, don't want to know about ECMO, don't want to know about chest tubes. I know I'll somehow put my head down and get through it, and on the other side I'll be grateful that I did and be stoked to be living life again.

My IV just beeped and I looked up to see that it's dripping out of the wrong bag! Two hours after being started and the medicine hasn't even begun—it's supposed to be finished!!! Now the morning IVs are going to be too early. UGH. But if I change the schedule, everything is going to be whacked, and I'm supposed to be going home tomorrow.

I wish I had Micah's ukulele here. I really felt happy when I was playing it. I felt calm, unaware of the passage of time. It was the middle of the night, no one was calling or texting, it was just me and the chords to some songs, my fingers practicing in order to get some muscle memory. I guess it's the closest thing I can get to a sport now. The movements of my fingers are just like the skills in volleyball or a swim stroke, and you have to do it so, so much before you become good at it. But there's pleasure in the effort of doing it, even before excellence.

6/3/17

I'm really pleasantly surprised by how nice my life is here. It'll sort of hit me by surprise, maybe when I'm hanging out with people from Bakery Living, or if it's a nice day in Pittsburgh and I have energy and we do something fun. But then sometimes it's a nice day and we do something fun and I still feel this malaise.

I just feel like life is passing me by. And I know it's not fair to complain about that because things could be SO much worse— I could be living in a hospital, instead of at Bakery Living and occasionally hospitalized. I could have no friends here and nobody visiting and no Jack. So I'm feeling grateful for all those things. And I am partly in control of what I do with my days, and I could spend them doing more productive things and whatnot. But I just can't shake these bad feelings.

Sometimes it feels like there's a hand inside my chest, taking my heart and squeezing it tightly so that it becomes hard to breathe for reasons completely unrelated to my lungs. And my heart will start to race and I'll feel this sense of panic. And I know this anxiety is new, and it's a growing problem. I'm just not sure what to do about it. I don't want to keep taking Ativan because, first of all, if I'm dependent on Ativan, that doesn't look good to the transplant team. And second, I think if I use Ativan a lot, then when I don't use it, I'm more irritable (I think that's a thing?). So I'm trying to relax and let it pass. Sometimes I cry, sometimes I watch TV, sometimes I write in this journal. But I feel like that solidifies this narrative—that I'm anxious and struggling and miserable. When really, that's NOT true most of the time these days; it's just that the times when it *is* true have a disproportionate impact on my perception of my life experience. And that's when I feel like writing.

6/13/17

Thursday night Jack came to town! I heard him come in at 1:30 a.m. and I hadn't been to sleep because I was lying there, tossing and turning. So I went into the kitchen to have a snack and say hi, and I scared him so badly, he jumped about five feet in the air! It was hilarious. We had a really good visit. It felt like things were back to normal with us after our heavy conversation. I think it was the fact that I'd finally unloaded the things that I was feeling upset about, and we talked through it, and then he got my anniversary card, which was really sweet, and he was very grateful about that and he really realized he needed to step up. And I know part of it was just that I was in a vicious cycle of anxiety where resentment was building and I was too scared to bring it up, and that made me more anxious, which meant I was even more sensitive to things he would do/say and make me more resentful and doubtful about our relationship.

So when he was here it just felt like we could have fun again and add good memories to the bank. Friday afternoon we got massages together, then we went to the patio to lie in the sun. I realized I really do love him and hope we have a future—and that a lot of my doubts are because I'm so unhappy with my situation.

6/25/17

It took me a second just now to think what month it is. Time FLIES.

I'm reading a few books now. Trying to feel more accomplished, and also to keep my brain stimulated. I'm reading *Watership Down* by Richard Adams, *Guns, Germs, and Steel* by Jared Diamond, and *All These Wonders* by Catherine Burns. It feels good to read, but I only do it at night. It's this weird thing where during the day I say to myself, "Pick up the book, pick up the book," and I know I'll be happy if I do, but there's this rebellious part of me that is like, "Fuck it, watch Netflix instead."

At the moment, I'm reading *Guns, Germs, and Steel* and it's 3:30 a.m. Can't sleep. Insomnia. Bo came to visit today. He and Michelle helped launch Lunges4Lungs, the social media campaign we're doing for transplant rejection. It's crazy that more attention hasn't been paid to this serious problem.

I'm reading about the origins of humanity and the divergence between African *Homo sapiens* and European *Homo sapiens* and the difference between Neanderthals and Cro-Magnons, and it's reminding me that I used to be intellectually interested in things, and that I used to have a spirit of adventure. The idea of going places used to excite me, not fill me with a sense of panic and dread. And I just want to COMMIT to myself that I WILL get that back one day. One day, after transplant, when every day isn't a struggle to survive, when I'm not aching and short of breath and nauseous and exhausted all the time, I WILL travel. I will appreciate wherever I live but I will also get out and see the world, knowing we don't have all the time in the world.

Caleigh has to be listed for a SECOND double-lung transplant. I can't believe it. It hasn't even been two years since her first one!! And she's had like three major health struggles since her first transplant, so it really seems like she can't catch a break.

7/8/17

Caleigh got rejected from Stanford for a second lung transplant. So now they're looking into coming to Pittsburgh. I hope so badly that it works out for them. I got a bad feeling about it when they suddenly discharged her from the hospital two days after telling her she'd have to stay inpatient until the next transplant. It seems as if they're giving up on her and they want her to spend her last days outside, enjoying herself. She has so much will to live, and I hate when centers are so utilitarian in their thinking; that's what led everyone to reject me, too.

7/17/17

I've been having a lot of small bouts of hemoptysis recently.

Because I've had to skip so many treatments lately, post-hemoptysis, I feel more short of breath and have had more tachycardia. My last blood work showed I'm low on vitamin A and now I'm wondering if maybe I'm low on vitamin K, too, and that's why I keep bleeding day after day?

8/3/17—Diane Shader Smith

At 8:30 the other night, I parked in a handicap space across the street from Millie's Homemade Ice Cream so we could get dessert—one of the simple pleasures Mallory can still enjoy as she is tethered to oxygen and at the end stage of her battle with cystic fibrosis.

When we were coming out of Millie's I saw that a tow truck had my car on it and was ready to drive away. I ran across the street and told the driver that my daughter was at Millie's and I needed to go get her as it's hard for her to walk because of her medical situation.

The driver said, "I don't care what your daughter has—you can only have your car if you give me $200." I said I didn't have that much cash on me so he told me I'd need to pick up my car at their impound lot. I told him I wanted to call the police because she has a valid handi-

cap placard and the proper paperwork but more important, if he took my car I wouldn't be able to get my daughter home and her oxygen tank was running out.

The driver was beyond nasty and again said he didn't care what my problem was. He started to get in his truck to drive off, so I opened my car door and straddled the seat so he couldn't move without hurting me. I called 9-1-1 and explained the situation.

The nice police officer who answered said to stay put and tell the tow truck driver that the police were on the way. I started crying when I was on the phone because I felt helpless. Mallory was with me by now, standing to the side, visibly upset about what was happening. She was connected to O_2 with two IVs running simultaneously. Anyone seeing her could only feel pity. That the driver ignored her and her situation left me stunned. And PISSED.

And then the driver just let my car down and drove off. I said thank you. But then three women and one man who were standing off to the side—a group I had noticed but not thought anything of—approached me. One said, "Don't thank him, we paid him to leave your car." I was STUNNED. I didn't know these people. I was deeply distraught and unsure what to do and they stepped in to help. They said they gave him $100 to go away and then refused to take any money from me, saying they know how many expenses we'll have after transplant and to use the money for my daughter.

I asked the woman who actually paid the driver what her name was and she said Jeanette Ware. I was in shock that people we'd never met before would do that for us. She said, "Welcome to Pittsburgh."

8/15/17

Feeling really good about things:

1. Even though UPMC only has one surgeon now, there's a chance I could get double-listed at Tampa—thank you, David!!

And my health is stable right now, so I am in a position to wait a while (fingers crossed it stays that way).

2. Jack came to visit this past weekend and it was wonderful. It was just the two of us, with neither of my parents here until my mom arrived late Saturday night. It was super low-key. Friday we had to stay in all day to wait for oxygen deliveries because my concentrator was broken, but it was lovely. Then in the late afternoon I tried to take a nap while he went to Whole Foods, and then he cooked an incredible dinner for us. He made rosemary duck, golden beets, yams, and tomato avocado salad. The next day was also really low-key, but we did get to take a walk and watch people play kickball at the park nearby. Things with us are so good right now, very loving and tender.

3. I'm on a mission to introduce new things into my life now that I feel like we're really going to be here for a while. I went to a yoga class for the first time in eleven months last night! My last yoga class was on Union Street in S.F., last September, the morning before I went back to L.A. because my grandma got diagnosed with cancer.

4. I'm going to try really hard to make the most of my time in Pittsburgh. I don't want to waste any days that I feel good. I want to have lists of things I love to do ready, so that on any day I feel good enough, I can do something!

8/22/17

It's Micah's birthday today! Wish I could be with him.

8/25/17

I GOT ANOTHER CALL FOR LUNGS!!! It was 7 a.m. and for some reason my phone didn't ring so they called my mom.

It's so funny because we had been despairing lately about how it felt like it was never going to happen and how we could still be waiting a year from now. And then the call came!! The lungs were increased risk and had to be on EVLP. Dr. D'Cunha reassured us that they don't use lungs if they're subpar.

I wonder if this call has anything to do with my score going up two days ago in clinic? You never want to decline, but when you're waiting for lungs, the sicker you get the more likely you are to get lungs.

Jack happened to be in Boston for work, again, which is an amazing coincidence. His going there has turned out to be my good luck charm! He said he would come here instead of going to Maine with his dad!!! Liana is coming tonight, too, so my mom won't have to wait alone. She doesn't want my dad to fly in until we're sure it's a go.

My mom took FOREVER to get ready. We got to the hospital four hours after they called us—the time you're allowed to take. Her reasoning was that the last two times we raced over they kept us waiting for more than ten hours and she hadn't properly prepared the house (whatever that means). This time she wanted to throw out trash, get laundry done, clean the house in case it's a go. By the time we were in the car, on our way to the hospital, we got calls from four different people, all asking where we were. One was a coordinator who was really nasty on the phone.

We didn't even go to a room on the floor this time, probably because we were so late. We just went straight to pre-op and they did the testing there. Everything was rushed and frenzied.

Jack showed up from Boston shortly after we got into the room. Everyone was talking over each other, and there were about five people surrounding me the whole time.

Eventually they took me into the O.R., so this time, I actually had to say goodbye to my mom and Jack for real. I was stressed-out in the O.R. They gave me two doses of Versed. A nice doctor, a cardiac fellow, put old episodes of *Friends* on her phone for me to watch. Eventually, Dr. D'Cunha came in and told me that the lungs were no good. I don't really remember what he said besides that. But he had talked to my mom and Jack for a long time about it so they shared the details.

It was a very young donor, a drug overdose. The lungs looked good and would've been a perfect match other than being hep C antibody-positive* but when they opened him/her (they don't tell you the gender) they saw the person had aspirated, and when they stress-tested the lungs, they started leaking fluid, which made it a no go. I guess EVLP is a good thing to rule out bad lungs.

9/10/17
We got another call!!!!!

TRANSPLANT

9/11/17—Diane
Nine-eleven is an inauspicious date for transplant but after twenty-four hours it's a GO!! Hoping God, karma, science or a medical miracle will help Mallory to the other side. Surgery could take twelve hours.

* * *

After a long night and a seemingly even longer day, Mallory's surgery was deemed a success by Dr. D'Cunha, who said her new lungs are pristine and the procedure went well. The next twenty-four to forty-eight hours are critical as that's when she is at risk from a surgical perspective. After that, the big concern is cepacia, *as this deadly superbug can still colonize the new lungs. We are cautiously optimistic!*

* meaning the donor had hepatitis C

As Mal lies heavily sedated on a ventilator, and we dare to dream about a new life for her, we shed a tear (many in fact) for the selfless person who gave our daughter the gift of life. We aren't allowed to know who provided the lungs so we throw our eternal gratitude into the universe and hope it finds its way to the family and friends of our beloved donor. We can't imagine their grief but will remain forever grateful.

9/12/17—Diane
Twenty-four hours post-op—Mal is stable and doing better than expected. Vital signs look good, no fevers, minimal sedation, less O_2 needed than anticipated, and, most important, tolerating the ventilator! Tomorrow she will go back to the O.R. so Dr. D'Cunha and his team can close her chest (left open so the lungs settle in). Hoping that by end of day tomorrow we will be over the surgical hurdle. Jack arrived late tonight!

9/13/17—Jack Goodwin
Diane texts me the room information. "CTICU Rm 18." That's cardiothoracic intensive care unit, room 18. Mark meets me at the elevators.

It is 2:00 a.m. when I see her, the first time since I left two and a half weeks earlier after the third dry run. Diane and Mark are exhausted so I'm on the night shift until 6:30 a.m., watching her.

She is sleeping soundly, faceup, about two dozen lines running across her body. The data lines run to an LCD screen behind her head, giving a full ten-second visual readout of seven body measurements. The rest of the lines pump in medicine. She has a ventilator hooked up to her lungs; a tube the diameter of a quarter goes in through her mouth. She won't be able to speak until she has it out.

She'd written short notes on a clipboard in order to communicate.

Her first question: "What medicine am I on?" She always likes to be in charge, especially of her own body.

I sit down and take it all in, getting used to the feeling of wearing a full-body medical gown, gloves, and face mask. Here we are, just us, in a moment we had both dreamed about—me since I met her, Mal for a lifetime.

The whirring of the medical devices makes the room strangely peaceful.

I'm beginning to doze off when her eyes flicker awake. She blinks a few times, slowly tilting her head to see if anyone is in the room. I stand up to put my face in her field of vision. She sees my figure in front of her, her eyes beginning to focus. She reminds me of a sloth waking up from a nap, but one who is also extremely high.

The recognition hits. Her eyes bug out and get huge, her arms rise up and start swinging about in the air. The LCD health monitor lights up in protest. Alarms blare and red warning lights flash.

"Whoa, whoa, whoa, heyyyy, Hi, yes, calm down. Chill, Chill, Chill . . . CHILL!"

Her heartbeat has jumped to 185. Her blood oxygen level starts to drop, her minimal energy stores used by all of the effort she is expending. She motions with her hands for me to get her pen and clipboard with paper.

"I have SO much to tell you!!" she writes.

I had thought she wouldn't be fully lucid for a few days. That clearly is not the case. I guess she is overachieving even now. So typical.

We catch up, our progress hindered by her lack of muscle memory for writing combined with her memory fog, which causes her to forget the topic of a sentence halfway through writing it.

I can't stop smiling.

She is alive, breathing, and the proud new owner of two lungs she was not born with.

"What does my chest look like?" she writes.

I tell her, "I could describe what it looks like, but there's a lot there, you sure you want me to describe it?" Her chest is still very much open but covered by bandages and her gown. She can't feel that part. Yet.

"Wait, describe what . . . ?" she writes, then stares blankly. She can neither remember nor see what she has just asked.

The sun rises and my shift ends as Diane comes back to take over.

9/13/17—Diane
Mallory had surgery mid-morning to close her chest and is now recovering in ICU. Watching her still sedated and connected to the ventilator, with tubes everywhere. I can hardly believe she's on the other side and that things went so well. Dr. D'Cunha (the AMAZING surgeon) and Dr. Plewski (the INCREDIBLE head of CF at UPMC) say she's surpassed expectations!! Still a long road ahead, but now that her chest is closed we can work toward the goal of getting her off the vent. It's been a VERY difficult few days in terms of pain.

9/13/17—Jack
I wake up in the apartment around 3:00 p.m. and make my way over to the hospital. Diane tells me it has not been a good day for Mal.

Now that she is recovering well, the doctors want to wean her off pain, nausea, and anxiety medication, enough so that she can control her own lungs for the first time—without the ventilator. The only problem is, when you take away the medications that make you not able to feel things, you start to feel things.

It's been hard but might get a whole lot worse before it gets better. I settle in for a long night on my second watch.

She has pain, nausea, confusion, nightmares, hallucinations . . . it's overwhelming for her.

"Do they have all of their knives? There might be one that got stuck behind my left lung."

No, Mal, they have all of their knives.

"My whole body feels like a squid."

I know, Mal, I know.

"Is there someone standing behind me?"

No, Mal, no one is there.

"Is the ceiling leaking? It's dripping all over me."

No, Mal, the ceiling is fine.

"Is my skull bleeding? Did they operate on my brain by mistake?"

No, Mal, your noggin looks great.

It's a long night. She calms down when we hold hands.

Somehow, we fall asleep.

Sometime later, she shakes me awake, asking for her pen and paper. With the most concentration I have seen so far, she writes a note that I will never forget.

"You have so far exceeded my expectation of what is possible for love."

I have gotten into the practice of reading the words aloud as she writes them, slowly, so she can rewrite words that end up being illegible. The full weight of the sentence does not hit me until she draws a heart.

I look up from the clipboard and into her eyes as she gazes back into mine.

Amid all of the chaos that we have become accustomed to, despite all of the hardship, Mal and I have survived, we are here, as a team, in the middle of the greatest battle Mal will ever have to fight, hopefully.

Red lights flash and alarms blare.

"WARNING! THE FOLLOWING LIMITS HAVE BEEN EXCEEDED: HEART RATE, BLOOD PRESSURE, OXYGEN SATURATION, BREATHING CADENCE," the screen reads.

Shit . . . shit, shit, shit!

Panic sets in. I realize I need to calm her down.

"I forgot to tell you, Cooper had a really big poop today." Cooper is her nine-pound dog, comprised primarily of white fluffy fur and love.

Her lips smile around the ventilator tube.

"Nice," she writes.

One by one the alarms flicker off. A nurse has rushed in, ready for anything.

"We're okay. Totally fine. Stellar, actually," I say.

The nurse looks skeptical, then leaves.

Mark comes to relieve my shift midway through the night, but I stay, unable to leave Mal.

9/15/17—Diane

MIRACLE—Mal got the ventilator out and is breathing on her own!! There aren't words to describe the moment you see your baby girl breathing with new lungs.

9/16/17—Jack

Now that Mal is off the ventilator, new sensations began to dominate her attention.

The first is thirst.

She is not allowed to drink but can suck on small sponges soaked in water. Swallowing is still too dangerous as she has a feeding tube inserted. It's much smaller than the vent tube, but aggravating to her throat, which is still tender. Though her hydration levels remain perfect, the sensation persists.

Finally, she has had enough.

Instead of asking for another soaked sponge, she asks me to come close. Talking is still challenging with such a tired throat, so all she can manage is a whisper.

"No. More. Sponges . . . Need. Drink. From. Bottle."

I tell her that's not allowed, that it's too dangerous. She grabs my medical gown with all her strength and pulls on me. Her eyes look manic.

"NEED IT. PLEASE," she whispers angrily.

I tell her that she will be okay, that we will get through this together. Mal glares at me, releases my gown, and slumps back into her bed, defeated.

9/17/17—Diane
Mallory's pain is unbearable, which tempers the joy we're all feeling now that she has new lungs.

9/17/17—Jack
More pain and discomfort continue despite Mal's progress.

> *It gets worse and worse through the day.*
> *"Why did I do this?" Mal asks, out of the blue.*
> *"What do you mean?" I say, confused.*
> *"Why did I agree to a transplant?" she asks.*
> *"Well, let's remember why," I say. "You had hours of treatment every day, treating but not curing a sickness that was only getting worse month to month, which was slowly but surely taking away your ability to live a happy and normal life with your family and friends. We knew a transplant would be hard—we knew it would be painful. But we also knew that the pain would be primarily condensed into your recovery period, resulting in the reward of a longer, healthier, more fulfilling life. Does that still sound like a good trade?"*
> *I wait for her to think about it as she stares vacantly into the distance.*
> *I feel thankful for a lot of things. Pride, joy, and exhaustion best describe the week.*
> *But transplant inflicts trauma. Mal has endured so much. Good thing she won't remember most of it . . . or so they tell us.*

9/19/17—Diane
UPMC transplant team continues to amaze . . . Two issues Mal was dealing with—vocal cord paralysis from intubation during surgery and a feeding tube that was stuck in the wrong place—have been resolved. Each molehill feels like a mountain until Drs. D'Cunha and Pilewski (and their stellar colleagues) work their magic. While pain is still unbearable for Mal, she continues to surpass everyone's expectations in terms of milestones. Today's victory—Mallory walked!!

9/21/17—Diane

Mal had her first hair wash in ten days, thank you, Eileen! HUGE smile, followed by tears when she realized her vocal cords still aren't working properly. Feeding tube can't come out until she can swallow, so she is now working with speech pathology and ENT.* Also acute and chronic pain teams are trying to find a regimen that will work. Today's activities include walking, swallowing, and breathing exercises. I have to take mandatory training to learn about post-transplant care.

9/22/17—Diane

Yesterday started with the expectation that things would continue to improve, but it turned out to be a very difficult day. When Mal felt she was at the breaking point, I reminded her that she has tremendous inner strength, a strong will to survive, and more love/support than she could possibly imagine. And to keep looking at the photograph of her diseased lungs to remember why she agreed to this traumatic surgery.

9/23/17—Diane

Today was GREAT! We heard blood cultures were clear (after they hadn't been), that her vocal cords are closing as they should, that Mal's walk was 175 feet!! We watched her blow 1,000 on her incentive spirometer (first days she couldn't hit 250) and her pneumothorax is improving.

9/24/17—Diane

Mal is still dealing with vocal cord paralysis and a chest tube still culturing positive for cepacia. The feeding tube and chest tube, which continue to cause major pain, should come out soon. The good news is Mal more than doubled her step count today—she walked a half mile!!

---

* ear, nose, and throat doctor

9/25/17—Diane

Today was all about swallowing. Mal continues to improve but can't get her feeding tube out until she can eat and drink. They say practice makes perfect. . . .

9/26/17—Diane

Each day brings new milestones—today Mal's feeding tube was removed and she walked stairs. Marveling at the MIRACLE!

9/27/17—Diane

Sixteen days after Mal's transplant, they are preparing for discharge (will take a day or two to get the home meds set up). Exciting but also terrifying as Mal still has a "swallowing disorder"—temporary, we hope—and is immunosuppressed, still with chest tubes, still in pain. They can't do a bronchoscopy to check for rejection because they don't want to risk stirring up cepacia. *Continue to think it's a miracle or a dream that I don't ever want to wake up from.*

9/28/17—Diane

Final chest tube clean-out, final PICC dressing change, and final instructions. Vitals and clinical assessment are good so Mal is cleared for discharge!! Still a long road to recovery—and a whole new set of meds—but getting out of the hospital is a major milestone. Used to sing "Somewhere over the rainbow there are lungs, and the dreams that we dare to dream we hope do come true." Now we sing ". . . over the rainbow, there WERE lungs." Mal, our dream came true.

10/2/17—Diane

Still so much pain but every day seems to be a little better. Mallory still does not have much of a voice yet and swallowing is still an issue. Hosted a dinner tonight for her friends in the lobby, which got her

*up and out of the apartment. Tomorrow we head to the hospital at
6:30 a.m. for post-transplant tests. Crossing our fingers that the last
two chest tubes come out as that will help with the pain. Mal washed
her own hair for the first time today. When she was changing her clothes
she noticed her chest was much smaller and asked if I thought they had
cut out some ribs. Hadn't heard that they did but wondering if her dis-
carded/diseased lungs were swollen and infected, making them enlarged.
One more question for the team tomorrow . . .*

10/6/17—Diane

*This week's activities for Mal included transplant clinic, blood transfu-
sion, magnesium, potassium and antibiotic IVs, physical therapy, CT
scan, X-rays, dressing change, and blood draws. Still lots of pain from
the last two chest tubes but we continue to hope for improvement. They
say all of this is part of routine recovery and she's doing well given that
she's twenty-six days post-op, twenty-four if you count from date of
chest closing.*

10/7/17

I haven't written anything since my transplant on September 11.
Typing with errors because I'm wearing a pulse ox.*

Want to remember getting the real call, Gaby coming in, sitting in the hospital for twelve hours. I told my mom while we
were waiting that if this wasn't the time, that I would need a
break. She looked at me with conviction and said it WILL happen
and you WILL get through it. I wasn't serious, of course, but it
was reassuring to see her so confident.

Night of surgery

Saying goodbye to Maria on the phone, crying. UPMC cam-
eras recording everything so that they can share my story.

---

* a device used to measure pulse and oxygen saturation

Heading into O.R., extreme anxiety. Not knowing if I would come out alive.

Will continue later, too tired to cover so much at one time. Pillboxes are crazy hard. Need to update the list:

POST-TRANSPLANT PILLBOXES

1. Domperidone QID
2. Calcite 900 mg BID
3. Misoprostol 200 mcg QID
4. Prednisone 15 mg QD
5. Bupropion HCL XL 150 mg QD
6. Ursodiol 250 mg or 300 mg BID
7. Voriconazole 200 mg BID
8. Bactrim (sulfamethoxazole) DS 1 tab TID
9. Biotin 1000 mcg QD PM
10. Prograf (tacrolimus) 4.5 mg BID
11. Levaquin 750 mg QD
12. Colace 250 mg BID
13. Simethicone 180 mg QID
14. Dexilant 60 mg BID
15. Mestinon (pyridostigmine) 60 mg TID
16. Minocycline 100 mg BID
17. Aquadeks 1 tab BID
18. Famotidine 40 mg QD PM
19. Melatonin 3 mg QD PM
20. Amitiza 24 mcg BID
21. Lopressor (metoprolol tartrate) 50 mg BID
22. Coenzyme Q10 100 mg TID
23. Senna 2 tabs BID
24. Gabapentin 300 mg QD PM
25. Dulcolax 10 mg QD PM

NOON

1. Domperidone
2. misoprostol
3. simethicone
4. Mestinon
5. Bactrim
6. magnesium 2 tabs

EVENING

1. Domperidone
2. misoprostol
3. simethicone
4. CoQ10
5. magnesium 1 tab

10/9/17—Diane

Mallory taped two TV segments today—ABC and CBS—about her journey. The simple act of cleaning up is a major milestone after you've been so sick that washing your face is a huge effort!! Each day seems to bring improvement, so clinging to the idea that slow and steady wins the race.

10/15/17

On my twenty-fourth birthday in 2016, I got the phone call from UPMC that they would accept me into their lung transplant program when I became sick enough to need one.

One month and one day after transplant surgery, I celebrated my twenty-fifth birthday with Pittsburgh friends and then spent the rest of my birthday weekend with Jack. But the recovery from this surgery has been more harrowing and more painful than anything I've ever experienced before, and it's a good thing I don't remember the worst of it. What I do know is that I had angelic family and friends who stayed by my side when I was on the vent, disoriented, in pain, and panicking, who reminded me why I chose to put myself through this: for the hope of a better life.

I never knew if I would live to see the other side of transplant, if any program would take a chance on me, but UPMC doctors did, and here I am. This year, instead of wishing for something else, I just sent my deepest gratitude to my donor, whose selfless choice to donate organs gave me the chance at a new life. My primary aim will be to make him/her proud.

10/20/17—Diane
Five weeks and five days after Mal's transplant they removed the final two drains and took out the remaining staples from the surgical site. Immediately after Mal said, "Today is the best day of my life!"

10/25/17—Diane
Oh what a difference a day makes. A day after being out with friends, we are in the ER with Mal about to get admitted. Double-lung transplant is not easy to recover from, so we're hoping it's just a bump in the road but Mal is still struggling with pain, nausea, loss of appetite, fever, speech, and swallowing issues. Just had CT, which revealed possible pneumonia; next will be a bronch to look for rejection.

10/27/17
Need to remember to write about these things:

Chest open, ventilator, million lines. ICU, writing notes, banging phone on bed—when the ICU kicked my dad out for shift change and I was terrified. Called my mom but couldn't talk because of the vent so I banged the phone on the bed rail to communicate my distress. She put Jack on the phone and he calmed me down until my mom could track down my dad and he came back. Subsequent fight with hospital personnel about insane rule of kicking families out of ICU during shift change, the time nurses are least able to be responsive because they are distracted giving reports to the next shift.

Indignities in ICU. Chest closing, starting to be lucid. Moving to second ICU room, then to transplant floor (7?). Blood infection, infected pleural fluid, infected port.

Extreme thirst. Fear, anxiety, panic attacks, worst pain of my life, wishing I were not alive for parts of it.

First time sitting in a chair. First walk. Difficulty of getting to the bathroom with four chest-tube receptacles and IV pole and me unable to walk or lower/lift myself onto/off the toilet.

Stacy visiting, then Eileen and Don, Natalie, Danielle, Maya. Kyle and Dave coming soon. Increasing step count each day. Being fed through nasal tube. Surgery on my vocal cords to plump them up so they can close, but failure. Thickened liquid diet with the threat of aspiration if I drink thin liquids.

Writing notes. Amazing doctors—Pilewski, D'Cunha, Kates,* Harano,** PA Marissa, many more. Great nurses.

Going home. OVERWHELMED. Wasn't ready at all, crazy pill organization with lots of help from my dad and Barb. Crying to Maya about how this was the hardest thing I had ever experienced, sleeping through most of her visit. Birthday and birthday dinner. Chest tubes staying in FOREVER. No showers. Scary weight loss, down to 110 (BMI less than 15). Forgot to write before, Sabrina's visit in ICU but too drugged to remember.

Pain management issues, nerve block solution for a while. How opioid epidemic is making it harder for legit patients to get what they need.

* the ENT treating Mallory's vocal cords
** one of the surgeons on D'Cunha's team

Strange reality of me feeling closer to Jack post-transplant because of how amazing he was, and him feeling more distant cuz I couldn't talk on FaceTime/phone as much cuz of fatigue/my voice being weak/being overwhelmed/having visitors.

Physical therapy and walking, speech not improving. Hope for 2018—travel, lots of time with friends and family, being healthy and hospital free, and writing my book!

Lots of visitors—Talia and Ronit, Becca and her mom Nancy, Ali and her parents, Nancy and Alan. Running around, lots of activity, fancy nice dinners to try to fatten me up, Ralph and Mary hosting us for cocktails, then fever on 10/25 and trip to ER and admission. Current insomnia. Tomorrow thoracentesis to culture and possibly drain the pleural fluid and make sure there isn't an empyema.* Then later on a bronch with biopsy to check for rejection/culture any infection that's there?

10/28/17—Diane
After having a good day yesterday, Mal spiked a high fever late last night, the hallmark of cepacia syndrome and cause for great concern. Drs. Pilewski and D'Cunha explained the challenges they face treating both infection and rejection.

Anyone who knows Mal knows she's got more inner strength than most, but it's hard not to be scared. On a happier note, Jack came today. If only love could heal . . .

10/29/17—Diane
The highs and lows of this weekend are indescribable. Simplest explanation for what's happening is that Mal has a worsening pneumonia, not

---

* a condition in which pus gathers in the area between the lungs and the inner surface of the chest wall

surprising given the cepacia *that's still hovering and the immunosup-*
pressants needed to keep rejection at bay. Treating for both is proving to
be impossible. We check Mal's temperature multiple times a day as she
can go from a high fever that leaves her listless and in pain, to seemingly
fine within the span of hours. There's reason to be hopeful as Mallory's
O_2, *BP, and HR are good.*

10/31/17—Diane
Mallory is facing post-transplant pneumonia with tremendous courage as
cepacia continues to wreak havoc on her fragile body. UPMC is using
every weapon in its arsenal to attack the moving target of symptoms.
Feeding tube is back in, antibiotics are layered on, and ancillary service
providers come to help with PT, swallowing, and walking. Pulmonary,
Transplant, and Infectious Disease docs confer and round daily as Mal's
case is "complicated." Cepacia is so resistant and virulent that no one
is talking about rejection. The silence is deafening.

It's been an exhausting week for Mal as she struggles to recover. The
days blur together with mornings incredibly difficult and afternoons much
better. Many medical minds worked together to devise a cocktail of drugs
that will keep the cepacia at bay. Morning vitals were cause for great
concern.

11/3/17—Mark
I found an online article about Tom Patterson's case, the first case of
successful phage therapy in the United States. I reached out to his wife,
Steffanie Strathdee, Ph.D. an epidemiologist, and the one responsible
for wrangling phages for Tom. After I explained Mallory's situation,
that her B. cepacia *was rearing up again and would likely kill her if we*
couldn't get it under control, Steffanie agreed to help.

She reached out to her network of phage researchers, those who had
helped her save Tom's life, and soon we were in communication with them.

11/7/17—Diane

Mal isn't getting better. Since there is no hope left from traditional, approved medicine, Mark asked Mal's doctor if he would help us pursue phage therapy. Dr. Pilewski said, "YES, but if we're going to do this, we need to do it now, as we're out of time." We are now working with UPMC, Adaptive Phage Therapeutics, the U.S. Naval Medical Research Center, Texas A&M, UC San Diego, AmpliPhi Biosciences, the University of Michigan, and the University of Alberta to find an appropriate phage treatment.

11/9/17—Diane

One week ago we had NO options left to treat Mal's pneumonia since her cepacia is resistant to every single antibiotic on the market—the same cepacia that was in her old lungs is back in her new, pristine lungs. But now we have hope as Mark is working with the doctors to get phage therapy for Mal. If I wasn't a witness to what transpired this week between so many doctors at so many institutions, I would never believe it could happen. Isolates have been sent to various labs and phages are being tested in different parts of the country and Canada. While not a sure thing, it's the single most promising treatment we can try to get.

Mark also found a drug made by the Japanese pharmaceutical firm Shinogi (not yet approved in the United States) that might be active against cepacia. We brought it to the attention of our team at UPMC, who told us they'd been actively trying to secure it but there wasn't inventory. Danny knows someone at the company so he is putting us in touch. But UPMC said we didn't need to activate this connection, as they had just secured a full treatment course for Mallory!!

In the span of five days we went from feeling hopeless to hopeful. It's been a totally overwhelming week with an endless cycle of multiple teams rounding, IVs, RT treatments, PT, swallowing therapy, procedures, and showering (a BIG deal). One of the hardest parts is getting those darn compression stockings on. Such a relief that Linda is here and took on that job!! I am so grateful she is here!!

11/10/17—Diane

Things took a turn, Mal is much worse, we're in final throes. Dr.
Pilewski will do what it takes to keep things going. Starting the new
drug today (Herculean efforts were taken to make this happen) and hop-
ing it will work or act as a bridge until they find phages. At Dr. Pilew-
ski's urging, we are asking family and friends to fly in.

11/10/17—Jack

Today is my birthday.

I wake up with a jolt to the sound of my alarm.

A single notification is displayed on my phone, showing that Diane
had called me not even five minutes before and left a voicemail.

I shoot up in bed, fearful that something bad has happened.

I hit the voicemail playback button and Diane's voice fills the room.

"Jack . . . if you're going to come, come now . . . (click)."

Fearing the worst, I call her right back. It's time.

On the way to the airport, Mal checks in with a text. "Good morn-
ing!! I hope today is wonderful and that this birthday is the start of an
amazing year. And I hate to put a damper on the day but I'm getting
moved to the Intensive Care Unit." She ends the text with a sad faced
emoji. Even as she was struggling for her life, she was thinking about oth-
ers. Quintessential Mallory.

When I ask Diane why the urgency to come, she explains that Mal
is at the end and it is time to call anyone who needs to be there. By 8:00,
I'm in the room, along with thirty others who have flown in to be with
Mallory.

11/11/17—Jack

Things are scary, as Mallory isn't turning around. Diane arranges for
all of us to stand outside Mallory's ICU room and take a picture smil-
ing. Intubated and drugged up, Mal scribbles: "Can't talk at all (sad
face) but so grateful that you are all here for the hardest part." She smiles,

so remarkable in light of what is happening. She is writing notes to everyone, thanking them for visiting. At one point, she gets tired and tugs on my sleeve, pointing to the paper and motioning for a pen: First she writes, "Can we be alone." I squeeze her hand and indicate yes. Then I ask the others to give us a moment. She continues writing: "Is everyone here because they think I'm going to die?"

This is a hard question to respond to. I steady myself and answer as calmly as I can. "We knew this situation was risky, so everyone just wanted to be sure," I say vaguely, knowing how stupid it sounds. But I am trying to follow Diane's lead. Her mandate, in fact. She has very clearly and unequivocally instructed all of us to stay positive. She has chosen to ignore the advice the doctors have been giving for the past week, which is to let Mallory know she is dying. Diane feels strongly that since Mark is on a mission to get her phage therapy, there is still hope. And Mallory needs hope to hang in there.

Mallory looks into my eyes, searching for the truth. After a moment that seems to stretch far too long but in reality is only a slight pause, she shrugs her shoulders, tilts her head, and nods.

11/12/17—Diane

Things are spiraling out of control. I continue to insist that no one tell Mallory she is dying. Mark and I agree that we want her to take her last breath thinking she is going to sleep and will awaken when the phages have done their job. She is terrified of dying and my response as a mom is to try to take away her fear.

11/13/17—Diane

UPMC is working its magic to keep Mal stable. One of the labs in Maryland has confirmed that they have at least two active lytic phages that should be ready for delivery (expanded AND purified) by Thursday. Mark is in high gear coordinating additional phage preps to maximize Mal's chances. Dr. Pilewski said she won't make it to Thursday.

Mark thinks we should have the phages delivered and administered in whatever state they are in. Mark called Dr. Robert (Chip) Schooley, the one guiding us through the phage therapy journey, to ask about stopping the growth/purification process and using whatever phage prep is now ready. Jack came up with the idea to split the not-fully-mature existing culture in two, so one could be ready to administer and the other would continue the growth/purification process.

Mark texted this new idea to Chip. Chip liked it, and passed it along to APT.

Mark and Danny talked to APT, who gave us an ETA of 4:00 p.m. Tuesday for the first phage preparation.

I sent urgent emails to Drs. Pilewski and D'Cunha asking if we could use the UPMC chopper since they use them for organ procurement. They said yes!!!!

11/14/17—Meryl Shader (Mallory's aunt)
It's the early morning shift and I'm sitting alone with Mallory, who rests fully sedated. It's not clear what she absorbs in this state but Diane thinks, as do I, that she knows we are there, so I keep my hand on her leg and believe she feels the presence of family. When I remove my hand to take photos of Mal's vitals, I explain to Mallory that I just need my hand for a minute to use my cellphone, that her mother loves her so much, and she likes to see the machines' readings.

I take photos every hour per Diane's request and send them to her, so that she can know the status of Mallory's O_2, the most important number she's tracking. Diane is trying to sleep in the apartment but hasn't been able to during this critical time. I hope the good numbers enable her to doze until it's time for the next set.

11/14/17—Diane
Just got word that the helicopter can't fly in current weather so they're sending Dr. Harano to Allegheny County Airport to fly by plane to

Frederick Airport, the airport closest to APT's lab. APT will be waiting to hand off the phages and then Dr. Harano will fly back to Allegheny and be met by an ambulance to deliver the phages. Dr. Abdel-Massih will be waiting at Mallory's to prepare the phages for administration.

11/14/17—Meryl

With the phages on their way, everyone is whirling about in such a frenzy of excitement that I am terrified the excess energy will affect Mallory's numbers. There has been a great deal of conversation about keeping Mal's room a calm, meditative space because noise and excitement appear to cause her numbers to go crazy. So as everyone else bounds back and forth at her doorway, bringing status reports, racing off to watch the helicopter that is delivering the phages to the hospital roof, I stay in the chair by her bed, and hold her hand. My voice is steady as I deliver a very long monologue, reminding her of the beautiful days to come after the phages do their work. And I try to describe a medical process I barely understand. People come in and out. I feel like a drill sergeant, reminding them to keep their voices low. "The phages are coming," I say, we all say. "The phages are coming, Mal. They're almost here."

11/14/17—Diane

We need a miracle.

5:10 p.m.—Dr. Harano is on the plane with phages in hand. Turns out he will be met by a helicopter to bring the phages to the hospital by 6:00 p.m. The plan is to deliver them into the trachea. Everyone in the ICU is on standby. . . . Dr. D'Cunha was instrumental in securing transport, Dr. Pilewski will deliver the phages through a bronch. My new favorite quote: Some superheroes wear capes, others wear stethoscopes!!

5:55 p.m.—THE PHAGES ARE HERE!!! Dr. Abdel-Massih takes the cooler to the lab to prepare the first doses.

6:00 p.m.—Dr. Abdel-Massih brings three syringes into Mallory's room, and delivers them to Dr. Pilewski. Dr. P empties one through a bronchoscope into Mallory's right lung, and then a second one into Mallory's left lung. He then administers a micro-dose intravenously. I ask Mark how long it's supposed to take, and he tells me that Tom Patterson woke up from a month's-long coma and recognized his daughter seventy-two hours after the phages were administered. Now there's nothing to do but wait for them to work.

11/15/17—Diane

Mal started desatting around 7:00 a.m. UPMC docs paralyzed her chest to keep her from expending energy fighting against the ventilator.

Mark, Micah, Maria, Jack, Meryl, Danny, Eileen, Stacy, Cindy, Ron, Jesse, Marissa, Mich, Nicki, and Tyler are here for Mal, with Susie fetching food for all of us as we stand by in a minute-by-minute race with time.

11/15/17—Jack

I have to fight to wake myself up when I first hear the phone ring.

It's Eileen. "You need to come to the hospital now."

I throw on some clothes and run straight to the hospital. At the entrance to Mal's room, I gown up and join Diane and Mark, who are stroking her hands and speaking softly to Mallory. Her playlist of favorite songs is on in the background. They see me, then step aside to give me time with her.

Mallory is on her left side, her body angled to encourage the flow of blood to her left lung, the one that isn't completely overtaken by pneumonia. The right lung is completely saturated.

I sit beside Mal, holding her hand, squeezing it hard. Her vitals are terrible and visibly dropping.

"Mal . . . I'm really glad I met you . . . I want to thank you . . . for making me a better man . . . I love you Mal . . . always."

I break down in the moment. I had only cried once this hard before, the night that Mallory's Stanford doctor had said she'd have a year to live.

Now here we are, fifteen months later, powerless. We had fought so hard—and she had come so far—but now she is slipping away.

When I leave the room to give others their chance to sit with Mallory, Dr. Pilewski takes Mark, Diane, Micah, and me aside. In the staff room, he informs us, in clear, simple language that irreparable damage has been done to her brain due to lack of oxygen. Mallory's identity—her endless wit, fierce love of others, and inner spirit—is gone.

In that moment, we know it is time to let her go. She has endured enough. Diane doesn't want to tell Mallory she is dying and makes the decision that our last words will be ones of hope.

Diane is resolute: "If anyone deserves to rest in peace, it's Mallory." Micah is sobbing. Mark is distraught. We walk back to Mallory's room and join Meryl, who had stayed with Mal while we left to confer with the doctor. Everyone else is in the waiting room so it's just family for the final moments. Doctors begin switching off the devices working so diligently to keep her alive. One by one, the whirs of each machine vanish.

Together we hold Mallory so she feels our love, each of us taking a hand, her head, a leg. We speak to her, saying, "It's okay to sleep. You have the phage, it's going to work."

11/15/17—Diane
Despite everyone's heroic efforts, our brave, beautiful, loving Mallory passed peacefully today at 4:52 p.m., surrounded by Mark, Micah, Jack, Meryl, Danny, and me. The phage therapy we got for Mal couldn't be administered in time to save her but she will provide a lung biopsy so that researchers can learn from her case. Our hope is gone but Mallory's memory will be a blessing forever.

PART SIX

I have a strong urge to do something more . . . to write something that will change people, that will have an infectious influ-
ence on the way they think and feel that will last. I want to
create a piece so moving that people are in disbelief. And I want
it to be like handing people a pair of glasses, giving them a way
of seeing something they didn't even realize they weren't seeing.

—MALLORY SMITH

11/18/17—Diane
Mal called herself a cockroach, saying, "CF keeps trying to kill me but I don't die." In fact, she knew dying was a real possibility and left this note:

WHEN I DIE:

When I die, the most important thing I want my parents to know is that everything I am (and all the things I've been able to do) is because of them. As a daughter, a granddaughter, and a sister, my relationships have always been lopsided, because I can never give as much as I take. I wish I could repay them for everything they've done for me. Everything my parents and grandparents have done since I've been born was with the single-minded purpose of keeping me alive and well and happy and motivated, no matter how much it meant sacrificing themselves. I've never felt like I could express how much it meant that they were willing to give and give without expecting anything in return; I'd write cards, buy gifts for the holidays and birthdays, but no gesture comes close to being big enough.

The tiniest moments have stuck with me in the most profound ways: that time my dad slept on a springy cot in my hospital room for the eighth night in a row, in hospitalization number twenty-something, and told me about how he felt when his own dad died (lost and lonely, like he had come untethered, all of a sudden lacking roots or a home); all the times my mom put my needs over hers and didn't pursue the illustrious career she, as such a smart and hardworking woman, could have had; the times my brother offered to do my errands because I hadn't slept or wasn't breathing well; the hours Grandpa and I spent listening to symphonies and chamber music string quartets, bonding over Bach and Beethoven; sunny days spent sitting on the beach with Grandma in Hawaii throughout the years, joyous because we were together and by the water; lazy hours passed in the kitchen with Maria, debating the merits of Catholicism and the existence of God, knowing that despite our wildly different upbringings we would always be connected.

The most important thing they must know when I die is that none of these moments are forgotten, and they all contributed to me becoming a person who feels the world is a good place. I could have been a bitter person, might have felt cheated by getting stuck with a chronic terminal illness, if I weren't born into a family that surrounded me with fierce love and unwavering support from my very first breath.

I hope to be remembered as a kind, honest, good-hearted person who worked hard and put others before herself whenever possible.

I would like to be cremated, and hope to be celebrated on the water, where I always felt most at home, and for my remains to live on there.

A big funeral party would be good, too, for those who are unable to paddle out or are not comfortable on the water. Overall, I want people to celebrate my life with joy for the time we had together, rather than mourning my passing.

POSTSCRIPT

by Steffanie Strathdee

I never had a daughter, but if I had, I would want her to be just like Mallory. People might find it strange that we never actually met, spoke, emailed, or texted. That's because the first time I heard about Mallory, she was two months out from her double-lung transplant, fighting for her life against a superbug—B. cepacia—that threatened to devour her new healthy lungs. All her energy was expended on living. And breathing.

In early November 2017, her dad, Mark, reached out to me through their family friend, Rebecca. I returned his call immediately and felt Mallory's anguish through her dad's voice. He and his wife, Diane, had heard about phage therapy a few years earlier, so they were excited to read the news that my husband, Tom, had been successfully treated for a superbug infection.

I learned about phage therapy when Tom's dire prognosis caused me to look into alternative treatments. Desperate to see if phage therapy could save Tom, I reached out to my physician colleagues at UC San Diego and to researchers around the world. Together, we launched a "phage hunt" to find phages that would match Tom's bacterium. At the eleventh hour, they found several matching phages and we obtained approval from the Food and Drug Administration to use it on a compassionate basis.

It worked. Tom's recovery was a watershed moment in the strange history of phage therapy and the story went viral. But could it be a miracle for Mallory? Mallory's family, her boyfriend Jack, and I pledged to do everything in our power to find out.

*I turned to Twitter, pleading to phage researchers around the globe,
asking if they had phages active against Mallory's nemesis,* B. cepacia.
*My message was retweeted 432 times. A colleague of mine at UCSD,
Dr. Robert (Chip) Schooley, who oversaw Tom's phage therapy, joined
in the effort. We also turned to the people who had helped save Tom,
phage researchers from Texas A&M and the U.S. Navy Medical Research Center, along with a new company that worked with them,
Adaptive Phage Therapeutics (APT). A researcher from Alberta, Canada, Dr. Jon Dennis, who responded to my crowdsourcing tweet, agreed
to assist, too. Mallory's doctors sent her bacterial cultures to all the labs
who had joined the phage hunt. The press picked up the story. Suddenly, the whole world was watching.*

*The wait was interminable. I knew what it was like, since I had
been there myself. I sent Mallory a plush phage toy to give her hope
while she was in the hospital. Mark, Diane, and I emailed and texted
one another, Chip, and the other doctors around the clock. We waited
only for a few days, but they felt like months.*

*The Dennis lab was the first to find a phage active against Mal-
lory's bacterial infection. They couriered it to APT's lab for purifica-
tion and expansion. While it was en route, the Navy found another
phage with activity against Mallory's organism. The team was ener-
gized. Just when it seemed that we were going to pull it off, Mark
called me at dawn one morning to tell me that Mallory had taken a
turn for the worse. Her doctors thought they could keep her alive, but
only for a few more days. The phages weren't yet scrubbed of all of the
debris that accompanies them. And the phages had yet to be "grown
up"—amplified—so that they existed in sufficient quantity to treat
Mallory for at least a few weeks. The lab techs had pulled multiple
all-nighters, but they were out of time. It was now or never; if we
didn't act now, Mallory would die. Jack, who has a Masters in Engi-
neering from Stanford but knew nothing about phage therapy, suggested that the existing phage preparation be split in two, with one*

part to be administered in its existing "dirty" state, and the other half
to be amplified and scrubbed for later use. It was an incredible idea that
no one else had thought of.

Mallory's family and friends were filled with hope when the phages
arrived. Friends who had flown to Pittsburgh to be with Mallory took
videos. Facebook lit up with hundreds of posts, prayers, and cheers. I
watched from afar with bated breath, knowing that my job as a "phage
wrangler" was done. It was the phages' turn.

Chip coached the Pittsburgh doctors on how the phages should be
administered, deciding they should be given intratracheally instead of
intravenously, as they had been in Tom's case. Mark suggested, and the
doctors agreed, that Mallory should also receive a microdose intravenously in the hope that intravenously administered phages might be
better equipped to reach their superbug targets. Every clinical decision
was agonizing.

By the time the first doses of phage were administered, Mallory was
no longer conscious. She received one dose intratracheally into each lung,
and the intravenous microdose. Then we waited to see what would happen. The next morning, as the doctors were preparing the second set of
phage doses, Mallory continued to deteriorate, prompting her doctors to
explain that her low blood oxygen level had persisted long enough to
cause irreversible brain damage. Mark and Diane made the most gut-
wrenching decision parents will ever make: to remove their child's life
support. The moment I got Mark's text that she had passed away, I was
overcome with a deep sense of grief.

A few days later, Tom and I drove from San Diego to L.A. for
Mallory's celebration of life, held at a school in the Smiths' neighborhood. The auditorium overflowed with more than a thousand friends
and family members who sang, read poems, showed pictures and videos,
and told story after story that reflected how special Mallory was. No one
wanted it to end . . . to face the fact that she was really gone.

After the service, I wove through the crowd to introduce myself to

Mallory's parents. When they embraced me, I knew that we had become family and would forever be bonded.

At the reception, I met Jack. The pain in his eyes was almost too much to bear. I told him how sorry I was, but no words could capture what either of us felt.

"You and Tom were our inspiration," he whispered.

"Mallory was mine. And still is," I responded.

After I gave Mark and Diane big hugs, Mark pulled me aside and reminded me of something he had told me when we first talked on the phone. Had it only been a month ago?

"When I first heard about phage therapy," he said, "I asked Mallory's doctors if we could treat her before she had her lung transplant, so we could clear her infection and give her new lungs a chance." I nodded. It made total sense. "But they had never heard of this treatment," he continued. "They thought it was too risky and dismissed it. I can't help but wonder if it could have worked."

Even in their grief, Mark and Diane knew that Mallory's death and experience with phage therapy could help others. They had a biopsy of Mallory's lung sent to the Navy lab, where it could be examined to see if anything could be learned to move phage therapy forward. Although Mallory had received too few doses of phage and they had not been adequately prepared, the Navy team was extremely excited to confirm that the phages had found their targets and had multiplied in Mallory's lungs! This microscopic piece of data offers insight into how to target phage therapy to treat future patients with CF and lung transplants.

Mark's idea stayed with me. I shared it with Chip, who in turn shared it with Dr. Doug Conrad, who directs the CF clinic at UCSD. "It's actually a great idea," Chip told Mark and me later. "I hope we can give it a try someday."

That day came just a few months later in 2018, when a twenty-six-year-old CF patient from L.A. with a multi-drug resistant Pseudomonas aeruginosa *infection came to be treated at UCSD because her infection had made her ineligible for a lung transplant. Chip and Doug presented her with Mark's idea. Did she want to try phage therapy? She decided to give it a chance. A few weeks later, her infection cleared. She returned to L.A. and was approved for transplant. Based on our experience with this patient and several others, in June, 2018, we launched the Center for Innovative Phage Applications and Therapeutics (IPATH) at UCSD, the first phage therapy center in North America. IPATH is in the planning stage for the first clinical trial of phage therapy among CF patients with multi-drug resistant bacterial infections.*

Inspired by Mallory's story and by my attempt to crowdsource phages, two young researchers, Drs. Jessica Sacher and Jan Zheng, took a bold step and created Phage Directory, a nonprofit database to help patients with superbugs find researchers to donate phages to their cause. The heroic effort to save Mallory's life sparked an international movement to propel phage therapy forward as a legitimate treatment for superbugs, a movement exemplified by the recent establishment of IPATH. Mark and Diane directed Mallory's Legacy Fund at the Cystic Fibrosis Foundation to make an inaugural grant of $100,000 to IPATH. As resistant strains of bacteria become more virulent and common, phage therapy holds out hope for a future cure when antibiotics fail us.

The most inspiring people are ordinary people who have done something extraordinary. Mallory's legacy as a fierce young woman, determined to "Live Happy" while overcoming every medical challenge she faced, will live on in the words she left behind in this book.

ACKNOWLEDGMENTS

by Diane Shader Smith

After Mallory passed, and I struggled to accept that she was gone, her journals were the best source of comfort. I spent time every day for many months reading and rereading her words. Laughing, crying, cringing, cursing, I relived her life from the time she was fifteen to her death at the age of twenty-five. Knowing Mallory wanted to share the difficult parts of her story and having her trust me to do so gave me the drive to pursue publication.

My paramount concern was timing: determined to publish within a year (to support our efforts to bring phage therapy from the lab to the clinic, and to offer her words as a source of comfort to so many who loved her), I enlisted my sister, Meryl Shader, to help edit the selections I had pulled to prepare them for publication. We went back and forth for weeks, discussing which entries to use and in what order. Her expert editing was instrumental in helping me get the draft ready. She would continue to provide insightful comments and her immersion in the project enabled her to propose the perfect title. I then sent Lilli Colton the photograph of Mallory doing a headstand on the beach and asked her to design a cover. She did a beautiful job. Micah Smith read the draft and provided feedback with all the TLC a loving brother could offer.

The next step was to find an experienced and dispassionate editor to provide an unbiased opinion. Jessica Carbino suggested

Claire Wachtel. I googled her and immediately knew she would be perfect. Armed with two computers—one with the original 2,500-page journal and the other with the working draft—I flew to New York. Claire and I holed up for three long days, not breaking even for lunch, with her asking questions like: *Can you pull an entry from the prom? Do you mind if we cut the piece on page 158? It reads just like the piece on page 245. Would Mallory's boyfriend, Jack Goodwin, be willing to contribute his memories to the book as well?*

I am grateful to Jack for capturing memories from the most difficult time and for providing a voice for Mallory when she could not speak. But most of all for loving my daughter.

Over those three days with Claire, her invaluable guidance helped me finalize the entries that would best structure a narrative arc. Claire had me meet with Richard Abate, the talented agent who presented the manuscript to Cindy Spiegel of Spiegel & Grau, an imprint of Penguin Random House. I am grateful to Richard for his direction, understanding, and care in placing the book in the hands of someone who believed so strongly in it.

Meeting Cindy was magical. Not only did she say YES to publishing *Salt in My Soul: An Unfinished Life,* but she did the final careful edit. Cindy offered suggestions while respecting the integrity of Mallory's writing, cutting only where necessary to strengthen its impact. I am grateful to her and to the entire team at Spiegel & Grau and Random House—Mengfei Chen, Tom Perry, Maria Braeckel, Barbara Fillon, Dhara Parikh, and Andrea DeWerd, among others—for all their work on the book and their thoughtful handling of a sensitive project.

Equally important was the proofreading team that that helped me review the final draft. In alphabetical order: Jack Goodwin, Eric Lax, Debra Sarokin, Meryl Shader, Mark Smith, Micah Smith, Ronit Stone, and Karen Sulzberger. I so appreciate their meticulous attention to detail.

Mark Smith, my husband and Mallory's father, was part of every conversation—sometimes listening, sometimes leading, always supporting.

I'm deeply grateful to each of the people mentioned above for their part in bringing Mallory's words to the world, and to everyone who helped make Mallory's important but too-short life happier and more meaningful.

ABOUT THE AUTHOR

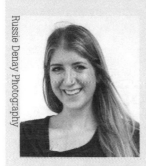

Mallory Smith, who grew up in Los Angeles, was a freelance writer and editor specializing in environmental issues, social justice and healthcare-related communications.

She graduated from Stanford University and worked as a senior producer at *Green Grid Radio*, an environmental storytelling radio show and podcast.

She was a fierce advocate for those who suffered from cystic fibrosis, launching the viral social media campaign 'Lunges4Lungs' with friends and raising more than $5 million with her parents for CF research through the annual Mallory's Garden event.

She died at the age of twenty-five on November 15, 2017, two months after receiving a double-lung transplant. Mark and Diane established Mallory's Legacy Fund at the Cystic Fibrosis Foundation in memory of their beloved daughter.

 faceook.com/MallorySmithAuthor

www.saltinmysoulbook.com

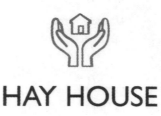

HAY HOUSE
Look within

Join the conversation about latest products,
events, exclusive offers and more.

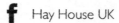 Hay House UK

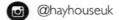 @HayHouseUK

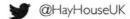 @hayhouseuk

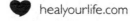 healyourlife.com

We'd love to hear from you!